# Dr. Kellyann's
# BONE BROTH
## Cookbook

# *Dr. Kellyann's* BONE BROTH *Cookbook*

## More Than **125 RECIPES** to Help You Lose Pounds, Inches, and Wrinkles

### KELLYANN PETRUCCI, MS, ND

RODALE

# RODALE
## *wellness*

*Live happy. Be healthy. Get inspired.*

Sign up today to get exclusive access to our authors, exclusive bonuses,
and the most authoritative, useful, and cutting-edge information on health,
wellness, fitness, and living your life to the fullest.

**Visit us online at RodaleWellness.com**

**Join us at RodaleWellness.com/Join**

Rodale books may be purchased for business or promotional use or for special sales. For information,
please write to: Special Markets Department, Rodale Inc., 733 Third Avenue, New York, NY 10017.

Printed in the United States of America

Rodale Inc. makes every effort to use acid-free ♾, recycled paper ♻.

Book design by Christina Gaugler

Photographs by Mitch Mandel/Rodale Images

Library of Congress Cataloging-in-Publication Data is on file with the publisher.

ISBN-13: 978–1–62336–839–5   hardcover

Distributed to the trade by Macmillan

2  4  6  8  10  9  7  5  3  1   hardcover

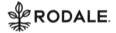

**RODALE.**

We inspire health, healing, happiness, and love in the world.
Starting with you.

rodalebooks.com

To Patrick, my life muse and forever friend. I'm so grateful to you for understanding me and my vision. No matter what coast, every meal I share with you is filled with intrigue, joy, and heart. I wish you a life filled with beautiful meals, travel, luxury, and love. #redhat #MrNYC

# CONTENTS

# ACKNOWLEDGMENTS

To Kevin: Thank you for showing me the world and how to appreciate the culinary masterpieces of more countries than I can count. Your contribution to my life has been priceless and I am forever grateful. I wish you the most decadent cup of hot chocolate from Café Angelina. #AfternoonsInParis

To my boys: Thank you for growing me up. Your support and love are my oxygen—and a big thanks for eating all those veggies and all that "blended stuff" when, let's face it, you really weren't into it. I'm so proud of you both.

To my parents, John and El: Your "Wild Italian Rose" loves you more than words can say. Thank you for letting me blossom and dealing with the thorns. It warms my heart to watch you never ever miss an end-of-the-day meal with each other for more than 54 years.

To my sister and two brothers: I will always remember our midnight cooking fiascos and family traditions. I wish you all a super-big bowl of hand-rolled cavatelli while watching our kids perform in this year's Christmas talent show.

To Jen, aka Jen Jen: Thanks for keeping me in line and being my rock for 25 years and counting. I'm not easy to "reel in," and I love and appreciate you . . . every day. You deserve the biggest bag of marshmallows in the world (you know, the healthy kind).

To the entire team at Dr.Kellyann.com: No way would there be a brand without your brilliance behind me. I honor you. I appreciate you. I thank you. I wish you passion and peace with all the meals you share with the ones you love.

To Cindy: You. Are. Incredible. Not to mention one of the most beautiful human beings in the world. You have never let me (or my books) down. I wish you and your hubby many more years and anniversary meals at #LaValencia.

To Alison: You might just be the most modest and humble person I have ever known. Thank you for loving this book. You are a blessing and a joy to work with. I wish you lots and lots of bone broth so you never get arthritis.

To Diandre: You are the strongest person I know. I admire your conviction so much. I always wonder . . . how is it that this young person has taught me so much? I love you and your style. A piece of you will always be with me. Thank you for saving me from more than just my fashion flops. I wish you a big handful of those M&Ms you keep on your kitchen counter . . . but promise me, just *one* handful.

To Elena: You give so selflessly. You love so fully. You always squeeze every morsel of your heart into everything you do. Your guidance and genuine enthusiasm for my vision have shown your true character. You pour beauty that goes way beyond your brushes into everyone you meet. I love all of our "catch-up" meals. I wish you so many blessings, topped off with a big slice of flourless chocolate cake. Yes, I said *flourless* . . .

To Robin: Thank you for believing in me. Thank you for going to bat for me, and thank you for trusting me. I don't know if you even realize just how amazing you are. I wish for every mug of your morning broth to warm your heart and soul and make you smile that beautiful smile.

To Keith: You are pure genius. I never know what you really see behind that lens, but it is always the best of everyone. I hope we have many more of our "it's a wrap" dinners.

To JJ: Thank you for teaching me to be a better entrepreneur. Thank you for teaching me to never say seltzer and to love squash. I have adored all our countless meals together—even our shakes with kale. I wish for you and Tim to have a lifetime of excitement over every meal, and every kiss, just as you do today.

To Celeste: Thank you for your high level of excellence and marketing prowess. I wish you many amazing memories and meals with your twin babies—and a belly so flat, you will rule the world.

To Peter: Thank you for having my back and telling anyone and everyone, "*No one* messes with Dr. Kellyann." I'm wishing you and your wife a night out at the finest Manhattan restaurant—with your cell phone off.

To Joe: Thank you for teaching me to love marketing, to be on time, and to always find a way. I wish you all the Paleo meals you love with all the beautiful people you surround yourself with, who admire and adore you so very much.

To Michael: Thank you for giving and giving and giving. I appreciate every bit of your genius. I appreciate you connecting and up-building everyone you meet. I wish you and Elaine a lifetime of love, and I look forward to many more of our Sanctuary meals.

To Neal, aka NS: Thank you for seeing something in me and telling me over and over again, "It *will* happen, I promise you." Knowing you are there for me means a lot. I appreciate your expertise and Hollywood know-how. I'm looking forward to what we'll uncover in the future. Cheers to your happiness and lots of picnics in the Cali sun with those kiddos!

To Iris: I am so grateful for that dinner I had at the Malibu Beach Inn that led me to you. Thank you for believing in me enough to encourage me along my path. You not only told me you believed in me—you showed me. I look forward to our dinners and chats at my favorite places, like Chateau Marmont. I wish you and your kids (doggies) lots of hearty, mouth-watering bones, bone marrow, and bone broth!

To all of my coaches and mentors over the years: Thank you for always keeping me in the spirit of contribution. I'm toasting you right now!

To Cesario: We have had the best time exploring L.A. restaurants. I appreciate every hidden treasure you've shared with me. From Ink to Little Door to AOC, every meal has been an experience. I wish you a warm glass of grappa topped off with a big scoop of that handmade coconut ice cream from Salt and Straw. You are a pure gentleman, my friend.

To all my patients over the years, my readers, and my viewers: You are my true teachers and the reason I get up in the morning. Thank you for having an impact on my life. I wish you a life of purpose and buckets of healing and regenerative bone broth.

To Rodale: Thank you for giving me yet another opportunity to shine. I appreciate all of you, and your wonderful work and collaboration in seeing this vision through. We made a great team. I wish you countless more NYT bestsellers and countless cups of broth!

# FOREWORD

As the chef and food stylist for *Good Morning America*, I'm passionate about helping home cooks create wonderful, no-fuss meals, while also promoting foods that help people stay slim and healthy. That's why I'm delighted to introduce you to Dr. Kellyann.

While food is my joy in life, it was once my problem. For many years, I struggled with my weight. Then one morning in January 2016, I met Dr. Kellyann at GMA and she changed my life.

There is something extraordinary about Dr. Kellyann. If you've ever seen her on TV, you'll know what I mean. She puts her whole heart and soul into everything she does. Like me, she's passionate about her message—and her message is that *you can transform your life with food*. I knew immediately that Dr. Kellyann had an authentic approach that I could follow and enjoy. She has hard science backing up her diet, which includes foods that I love and frequently use in my own kitchen. Her low-carb approach with the "elixir" bone broth is all so doable, and I felt inspired to begin my own transformation.

I decided to give the whole thing a try. I fell off the wagon a few times, but I got right back on. I knew that I could stick to this diet, and I did.

The results of my Bone Broth Diet thrilled me. My extra pounds started falling off, I had energy all day, and I felt *happy* again. In addition, I knew that I had the tools to maintain my success. I have a demanding job, a family, and a full life, and being slim and healthy is empowering me to enjoy all of them to the fullest.

What's more, the Bone Broth Diet really got my creative juices going! The foods on this diet are natural, vibrant, and luscious—nothing like the no-fat, no-taste foods on most diets. As a professional chef, I love the beautiful proteins, fats, fruits, and vegetables I can cook with on this diet. I've even contributed a few recipes to this book myself.

If you're ready to lose your own extra pounds, you're holding the solution in your hands right now. This cookbook is loaded with simple guidelines, practical tips, meal plans, shopping lists, and more than 125 recipes you're going to love. In addition, it's infused with Dr. Kellyann's generosity, spirit, and optimism. Let her guide your own transformation, just as she guided mine!

*Karen Pickus*
*Chef/Food Stylist, Good Morning America*

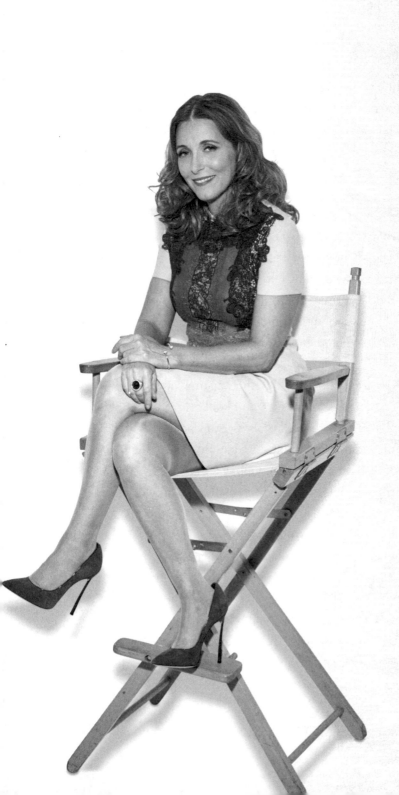

# INTRODUCTION

# *It's Your Time to Shine—Join the Revolution!*

YOU KNOW WHAT I did last year? I started a revolution.

I'm not talking about one of those marching-in-the-streets-with-banners revolutions. Instead, I started a *weight-loss and anti-aging* revolution. It's the Bone Broth Diet Revolution, and it's taking the world by storm.

Hundreds of thousands of people are now part of my revolution. Collectively, they've lost millions of pounds.

So—what's the Bone Broth Diet Revolution all about? It's about . . .

- Losing weight and taking years off your face by eating *real, delicious, awesome food*—not dry toast, skim milk, and egg whites.

- Eating like a real person, not a machine. No counting carbs, calories, or fat grams, or weighing your food on a scale.

- Getting rid of fake foods that make you sick—from soy Frankenfoods and fat-free "health" foods to additives, preservatives, and artificial colorings.

- Realizing that *your weight gain isn't your fault*—it's the fault of dangerously misguided advice from so-called nutrition experts who've caused the Western world's epidemics of obesity, diabetes, and diseases of aging.

- Discovering that when you know the truth about food, *you can take control of your weight—forever*. No more yo-yo dieting. No more hunger. No more cravings. No more food obsessions.

What qualifies me to lead this worldwide weight-loss and anti-aging revolution? I'm a naturopathic physician and certified nutritional consultant with more than 20 years of clinical experience, and my specialty is *transforming* people.

As a concierge doctor to celebrities in Hollywood and New York, I show top stars how to look flawless on stage and on screen. And in my clinical practice in Michigan, I work with everyone from slightly overweight people to desperately ill men and women who need to lose weight quickly to save their lives.

So believe me: I know what works. I'm not like most doctors, who are satisfied with a 10 percent success rate for dieters. My goal is *100 percent success.* If you'll commit to my diet, I'm going to take that extra weight off you.

And you know what else I'm going to do? I'm going to smooth out your wrinkles, taking years off your face. And I'm going to make you feel younger and healthier than you've felt in years.

In short, I'm going to transform you—and I'm going to do it in just 21 days.

That's a big promise, I know. But I have a track record of thousands and thousands of successful weight-loss and anti-aging transformations to back it up. What's more, I have hard data.

Before publishing my previous book, I conducted three trials in three different cities, conducted by three different clinicians. Here are the results after participants spent 21 days on the diet:

- They lost up to 15 pounds and 4 inches in their measurements.

- Their wrinkles and "double chins" diminished, their skin tone became more even, and their acne healed.

- They felt healthier. Two participants no longer required insulin after the diet, one was able to significantly reduce her dose, and another's shingles cleared up.

- They slept better.

- They felt better emotionally. As one participant put it, "I feel happy again."

Since my book came out, I've received thousands of emails every week from men and women who report their own transformations. They're slimmer, healthier, and happier—and they love how their skin looks.

If you too want to become a part of this revolution, come on in! In the next four chapters, I'll tell you exactly how the diet works. I'll explain why the magic lies in the power of bone broth—my liquid gold. I'll tell you how to keep those extra pounds off forever once you lose them. And then I'll share more than 125 *amazing* recipes that are so luscious, you won't believe you're on a diet.

Welcome to the Bone Broth Diet Revolution!

# PART 1

# HOW THE BONE BROTH DIET WORKS

If you read my earlier book, *Dr. Kellyann's Bone Broth Diet,* you already know the why's and the how's of my diet—so feel free to skip right to the recipe section.

If you're new to my diet, the next few chapters will tell you everything you need to know. In Chapter 1, I'll talk about why this diet works while other diets fail. In Chapter 2, I'll tell you how to follow the diet, step-by-step. In Chapter 3, you'll learn all about the "yes" and "no" foods on the diet, and Chapter 4 will show you how to make meal planning a breeze.

Let's get started!

## CHAPTER 1

# Why My Diet Is Different—And Why It *Works*

**HAVE YOU TRIED DIET** after diet, only to wind up frustrated and actually *gain* weight?

If so, trust me—you're not alone.

Every year, I see hundreds of people just like you in my office. By the time these people hear about me, many of them are desperate. They're overweight, they're unhealthy, and they look and feel years older than they are.

These people have tried diet after diet. They've dutifully counted calories, calculated fat grams, and weighed portions. And instead of losing their extra pounds, they weigh more than ever.

I call myself the "last-chance doctor" because I'm often their last hope. I can't fail them like their previous doctors did.

So I *don't* fail them. Instead, I show them how to take their extra weight off easily . . . and keep it off *permanently*.

And there's another way I'm different from their earlier doctors. When I talk with my patients about their weight problems, I don't tell them, "It's your fault."

You know why? Because if you're struggling with a weight problem, it's *not* your fault. Here's why.

## HOW THE "EXPERTS" MADE YOU GAIN WEIGHT

Before I tell you how to take off your extra pounds, I need to start at the beginning. So here's my question: What made you gain weight in the first place?

Here's the deal. It's not greed or low willpower. It's *bad advice*.

If you're like most people, you've spent years obediently eating what nutrition "experts" told you to eat: sandwiches, wraps, and mounds of pasta. Bowl after bowl of cereal. Margarine and heavily processed seed oils like canola oil. Soy burgers and other soy "Frankenfoods." Egg substitutes. Sugary nonfat yogurt loaded with artificial colors and flavors. Chemical sweeteners created in a laboratory.

What's the result?

- You're constantly spiking your blood sugar with high-carbohydrate foods. This causes your body to release more insulin—and *insulin lays down fat*. Worse yet, your cells eventually become resistant to this insulin overload and start slamming the door on insulin and the sugar it's carrying (a condition called *insulin resistance*). As a result, this sugar gets turned into fat and goes right to your belly. In addition, insulin resistance causes you to crave more carbs, creating a vicious cycle.

- You're making your gut sick. The trillions of microbes in your intestines play a *huge* role in determining how much you weigh. Feed them food they're not genetically wired to use—from massive amounts of soy to gut-altering pseudo-foods like sucralose—and you have an unhealthy ecosystem. This leads to body-wide inflammation (I'll talk more about this later) that *packs on* the pounds.

- You're robbing your body of the natural, real foods you need to keep your cells glowing, your hormones optimized, and your metabolism running on high. As a result, you're never truly healthy—and you keep gaining weight.

With millions of people following this bad advice, is it any surprise that we're currently experiencing an epidemic of obesity and diabetes? Yep . . . this is my shocked face.

## WHY CRAVINGS AREN'T YOUR FAULT EITHER

Now, let's talk about something else: those uncontrollable cravings you get for junk foods like doughnuts, pizza, french fries, and cupcakes.

I'm betting your doctors tell you that resisting these cravings is simply a matter of increasing your willpower. (They love to lay guilt trips on you, don't they?) But guess what: There are biological reasons for these cravings—and again, the diet that "experts" prescribe is largely to blame. Here's a look at two key reasons why it's hard to resist the siren song of that junk food.

## 1. Leptin resistance

Leptin is a hormone your fat cells use to communicate with your brain about how much energy you need. High levels of leptin make you feel full, while low levels make you feel hungry. That's why I call leptin your hunger trigger.

That's pretty straightforward, right? But here's where things can start to go wrong.

If you eat a diet loaded with high-carb foods—including so-called healthy foods, like whole grains, pasta, and brown rice—you can develop *leptin resistance* (similar to the insulin resistance I just talked about). These foods cause your leptin levels to rise, and eventually your cells compensate by becoming insensitive to leptin.

When this happens, your cells no longer hear leptin's message that you're full. So even if you don't really need to eat, you experience deep-down cravings—and you're genetically wired to respond to these cravings by seeking high-calorie foods.

## 2. Sugar addiction

If you eat a diet that's high in sugary foods, you can actually suffer physical symptoms when you go without them. That's because sugar is addictive.

You may be thinking, "Seriously, Kellyann? Isn't *addiction* a pretty strong word?" But it's no exaggeration. Think about this: Rats in a maze will choose a path that leads to Oreos as frequently as a path that leads to cocaine, and the Oreos have an even stronger effect than cocaine on a part of the rats' brains that's linked to addiction.[1] Moreover, animal studies show that sugar produces three symptoms consistent with addiction: cravings, tolerance (so you want more and more), and withdrawal.[2]

Now, let's talk about where the sugar in your diet comes from. Sure, some of it comes from candy and cupcakes. But if you're eating the way most "experts" tell you to eat, a large amount of it is coming from *the foods these experts recommend*. For instance, two slices of whole wheat bread contain more sugar than a candy bar. And nonfat yogurt sweetened with high-fructose corn syrup is a sugar bomb. When you eat foods like these constantly, you strengthen the Sugar Demon's grip on you.

## WHY MY DIET MAKES YOU SLIM

As you can see, the typical diet that "experts" prescribe is a quadruple whammy. It's heavy in carbs, raising your levels of fat-promoting insulin. It's high in foods that damage your gut, leading to inflammation—the biggest cause of weight gain, as I'll explain later. It's poor in nutrients that keep your body glowing with health. And it leads to leptin resistance and sugar addiction, both of which make it harder for you to resist the temptation to eat sugary junk foods.

So it's time to say goodbye to that diet and do something that *works*. That something is my Bone Broth Diet. I've used this diet to help hundreds of thousands of people around the world lose weight and de-age their bodies.

Why does my diet work when others fail? Because I have two secrets: fat-melting foods and my "liquid gold." Here's a look at each one.

### Secret #1: My fat-melting foods

My diet centers around real foods—the foods we're genetically engineered to need. When you eat these foods, it is simply *natural law* that you will get slimmer and healthier.

Here is what these foods do:

1. **They heal inflammation.** These foods are *loaded* with anti-inflammatory nutrients—and reduced inflammation equals a slimmer, younger-looking you. (I'll tell you why shortly.)

2. **They're low in carbohydrates.** When you eat fewer carbs, your blood sugar drops. This means you generate less insulin. Your insulin resistance starts to disappear, so you deposit less belly fat. In addition, your cells become sensitive to leptin, so you no longer crave food when you're full.

3. **They're lipotropic.** Lipotropic nutrients carry fat away from your liver and help you break it down and metabolize it. On this diet, many of the foods you'll be eating are loaded with choline, which is the body's main lipotropic substance.

4. **They're rich in healthy fats that nourish your body and skin.** I want you to drive a stake into the heart of the "fats are bad for you" myth. Healthy fats make you *lose* fat—and they're fabulous for your skin.

5. **They scrub your cells clean.** Right now, if you've been eating a typical diet, your cellular matrix—the "sea" in which your cells swim—is clogged and acidic. The clean, nutrient-dense foods you'll eat on this diet are brimming with detoxifying nutrients that will make your cells vibrant and young again.

6. **They regulate your hormones.** These real foods will help bring *all* of your hormones—not just insulin and leptin—into balance. As a result, you'll see changes in everything from your skin to your energy levels. By the way, one result that patients report all the time is what I call tiger blood. Let's just say—ahem— that you're likely to feel like a teenager again in more ways than one!

7. **They end your sugar cravings.** By satisfying your hunger in healthy ways, these foods empower you to break free from your sugar habit.

When you swap out the foods that are making you fat and sick for these natural, nutrient-loaded foods, you're going to see amazing results. The pounds will fall off, your belly fat will begin to vanish, your skin will look younger, and you'll feel better than you have in years.

In addition, these foods are *delicious*. You're going to look forward to your meals, rather than dreading them. You may even feel a little sinful when you eye your gorgeous plates—that is, until you see your muffin top and your wrinkles melting away.

## Secret #2: Painless mini-fasts with the magic of "liquid gold"

On my diet, you're going to do "mini-fasts" two days a week. (Don't stop reading—I have a *painless* way for you to do this, and I'll share it with you in just a few paragraphs.)

Mini-fasts are a part of my diet because fasting is the quickest way to strip pounds off your body. It lowers your insulin levels, ramping up fat burning. It increases your levels of human growth hormone, which burns fat and builds lean muscle. It cleanses your cells, removing the debris that makes them sluggish. And it heals chronic inflammation—the biggest key to fast, permanent weight loss.

In addition to these benefits, fasting creates a huge calorie deficit. While my diet isn't a calorie-counting diet, cutting down on your overall calories two days a week will burn your fat stores *rapidly*.

So if you're serious about losing weight quickly, fasting needs to be part of your plan. You can do this diet without the fasts, but the pounds will come off more slowly.

Now, I know you're still wondering . . . how can fasting be painless? Well, here's the secret:

*Bone broth.*

Bone broth is what makes this diet different from any other diet you've tried. Of all the foods I want you to eat, *this is the most crucial one*. It's the magic elixir that burns off fat, smooths your skin, and gives you the power to fast without fear.

If you're new to bone broth, it's a rich, flavorful broth made from meat, poultry, or fish bones that you cook for hours until they literally start to melt, releasing deep nutrition. It's this healing nutrition that gives my diet superpowers.

I know it may be hard to believe that one of the world's simplest and oldest foods holds the key to losing your extra pounds and erasing your wrinkles. These days, we're trained to believe that healing comes from a pill or surgery—not from something as basic as food. But there are three reasons why this "liquid gold" will transform your body. Here's a look at each of them:

1. Bone broth fills you up and eliminates cravings.
As I've just said, you're going to do bone broth "mini-fasts" two days a week on this diet. These mini-fasts are the key to rapid weight loss, because fasting takes pounds off like *crazy*.

The downside, of course, is that regular fasting is hard—in fact, far too hard for many people. Regular fasting can make you hungry, shaky, and desperate for food.

However, on my diet, you're not going to be hungry on your mini-fasting days. That's because you're going to drink delicious, healing bone broth all day. It's my secret to pain-free fasting!

If you haven't tasted bone broth, believe me: It's nothing like that watery stuff in a can. It's rich and comforting, and a cup will fill you up for hours. Our bodies crave bone broth's deep nutrition, so it satisfies us on a cellular level.

Just how tasty and satisfying is bone broth? Classy restaurants in New York and

Hollywood are selling it these days for $9 a mug. In fact, there are trendy bistros that sell nothing *but* bone broth—and they can't keep up with the demand. So trust me: Bone broth isn't just healthy, it's fabulous.

2. Bone broth melts off your extra pounds by healing chronic inflammation.
In addition to being a delicious drink, bone broth is one of the world's most powerful healing foods. In fact, cultures around the world have used it for centuries as a medical treatment. Here's why:

- It's rich in glycine, a powerful anti-inflammatory amino acid.
- It's filled with glucosamine and chondroitin, which heal your joints.
- It's loaded with gelatin, which soothes gut inflammation.

This last point—the gut-healing power of gelatin—is so important that I want to talk more about it right now. I mentioned earlier that sick gut leads to chronic inflammation and weight gain, and now I want to take a minute to explain why.

Here's the story. Your gut is home to an entire ecosystem called your *microbiome*. (I like to say that you're a "big bag of bugs.") The microbes in this ecosystem do everything from keeping your immune system in check to metabolizing your food and synthesizing key vitamins and hormones.

When your gut has the right numbers and kinds of these bugs, you're in good shape. Your gut is glowing, and your level of inflammation is low.

But what happens when you have the *wrong* kinds and numbers of gut bugs? When your gut becomes unbalanced, things can go downhill really fast.

Unfortunately, the modern world is cruel to your microbiome. A standard diet high in carbs, sugar, and artificial chemicals and low in critical nutrients suppresses beneficial bugs while allowing bad bugs to thrive. Antibiotics kill off swaths of your beneficial microbes. Stress, toxins, a lack of exercise, and drugs like NSAIDS and antacids create an unhealthy environment for them.

When these culprits cause your gut to become unbalanced, bad things happen. The microbes in your gut start cranking out toxic chemicals that inflame your intestinal wall. Normally, this wall is a fortress—but when it becomes inflamed, holes open up in it. These holes let toxins and undigested food escape into your bloodstream, where they don't belong.

# Is This Diet Right for You?

If you want to lose weight, look and feel younger, and have the energy of a teenager, the answer is yes! I have just a few cautions:

- If you're pregnant, wait until you have your baby and finish nursing before starting the diet.
- If you have type 2 diabetes, work closely with your doctor to make sure you adjust your medications correctly as the diet lowers your blood sugar.
- If you have any chronic health conditions, get an okay from your doctor before starting the diet—and ask if your fasting days will affect your medications.
- If you're getting over an injury or illness, wait until you're well before starting the diet.
- If you have a history of an eating disorder, make sure your doctor gives you the okay to follow this diet.
- If you're under 18, be sure your mom or dad checks with your doctor first.

Still trying to decide if the Bone Broth Diet is right for you? Take the Bone Broth Diet Quiz on the Resources page on my Web site, bonebrothdietbook.com/resources.

---

This invasion from the gut sets your immune system permanently to "on." It calls out warrior cells and sends them into battle, even though there's no enemy to fight. Instead, these warriors target your own cells, poisoning them with toxic chemicals. Basically, it's friendly fire.

Soon, inflammation spreads throughout your entire body. It's like a forest fire that never goes out. We now know that this inflammation is the *leading cause of obesity*. It sickens your cells in ways that cause you to put on pounds (especially around your belly), and in turn, this extra fat cranks out inflammatory chemicals. It's a vicious cycle, and it causes you to gain more and more weight each year.

So if you want to battle inflammation, the place to start is *in your gut*. Build a glowing gut, and you will have a rock-solid intestinal wall. Toxins will stop escaping from your gut, your immune system will stand down, and your inflammation will vanish.

The biggest secret to this healing is bone broth. Bone broth is rich in gelatin, which coats and soothes your gut, bathing it in anti-inflammatory nutrients that put out the fire inside you.

To help you understand gelatin's healing power, here's a good analogy. Did you ever rub aloe vera on a bad sunburn to soothe and heal your skin? Well, right now, your gut has the same level of heat—that is, inflammation—and this heat is what's making it leaky and letting toxins escape to inflame your entire body. Gelatin soothes and heals your gut, extinguishing those flames.

By the way, bone broth doesn't just help heal your gut; it helps heal your joints as well. The glucosamine and chondroitin in bone broth are the same nutrients many doctors prescribe for joint pain—and a recent study showed that these nutrients can be as effective as Celebrex in treating knee osteoarthritis.[3] This is an added benefit that my patients love.


3. Bone broth takes years off your skin.
If you're a veteran of low-fat and low-calorie diets, you know that they make you look old, wrinkly, and washed out. That's because these diets pull essential nutrients out of your skin cells.

On my diet, however, the *opposite* is going to happen. Why? Because bone broth is loaded with the building blocks of collagen. It's like mainlining collagen directly to your skin cells. It erases fine wrinkles, giving you younger, firmer skin.

Better yet, unlike Botox, bone broth has *lasting* effects. Botox only paralyzes muscles to prevent wrinkles; it can't rebuild your skin and make it look younger. Bone broth, however, builds strong skin from the inside out. One comment I hear over and over again from people on my diet is, "My friends keep asking me if I've had work done."

As a bonus, research shows that collagen peptides protect your skin from sun damage.[4] So in addition to erasing your wrinkles, bone broth helps stop new ones from forming. How great is that?

## ARE YOU READY FOR YOUR OWN TRANSFORMATION?

Now you can see why I call bone broth *liquid gold*, and why I give it the starring role in my Bone Broth Diet. When you combine the delicious, fat-melting foods on this diet with easy bone broth mini-fasts, you will take weight off like crazy—and people won't believe how amazing your skin looks.

So there's only one question left: Are you ready to join my Bone Broth Revolution?

Are you ready to get rid of your extra pounds—fast? Are you ready to erase your wrinkles and heal your joints at the same time? And are you ready to learn about my 80/20 diet, which will empower you to keep your extra pounds off *forever*—with no more yo-yo dieting?

If so, here's all I'm asking: Give me three weeks, and I'll give you the slim, energetic, younger-looking body you deserve.

Let's get it done!

## CHAPTER 2

# The Basics of the Bone Broth Diet

IN THIS CHAPTER, I'M going to tell you all about doing the Bone Broth Diet. In addition, I'm going to tell you about my 80/20 maintenance plan, which will keep your extra pounds off for good. I'll even tell you what to expect on the diet, day by day.

But before we get started, I want to tell you three things about this diet that I think will make you very, very happy—especially if you're a veteran of standard diets. Here they are:

- On my diet, you won't need to count calories, carbs, or fat grams—and you can stick that food scale in the cupboard. That's because I'll teach you how to select perfect portions naturally and easily.

- You also won't need to eat tasteless diet foods like puffed wheat, dry rice cakes, or runny fat-free salad dressing. Instead, you'll eat full plates of mouthwatering, restaurant-quality food. (One comment I love hearing from people following my diet is: "I made a three-course meal for company, and they demanded the recipes!")

- Most importantly, you won't ever need to be hungry, even on your mini-fasting days. I don't believe in suffering on a diet, because it's simply *not necessary*.

In short: no weighing or measuring, no eating foods that taste like cardboard, and no starving.

Now, let's talk about how my 21-day diet works. Five days a week, you'll eat three full meals and two bone broth snacks. Then, on your mini-fast days, you'll have five or six meals of bone broth—or you can substitute a light meal for the last cup of broth.

Here's a closer look at how your mini-fasting and nonfasting days will work.

## HOW WILL YOUR MINI-FASTING DAYS WORK?

I recommend picking nonconsecutive days—for instance, a Sunday and a Wednesday—for your mini-fasting days. Here's an example.

# Becky's Diet

Remember: You can pick any 2 nonconsecutive days for your fast days.

| SUN | MON | TUES | WED | THURS | FRI | SAT |
|---|---|---|---|---|---|---|
| Mini-Fast Day | Nonfasting Day | Nonfasting Day | Mini-Fast Day | Nonfasting Day | Nonfasting Day | Nonfasting Day |
| 6 cups of bone broth (or 5 cups plus a 7 p.m. snack) | 3 meals of "yes" foods plus 2 bone broth snacks | 3 meals of "yes" foods plus 2 bone broth snacks | 6 cups of bone broth (or 5 cups plus a 7 p.m. snack) | 3 meals of "yes" foods plus 2 bone broth snacks | 3 meals of "yes" foods plus 2 bone broth snacks | 3 meals of "yes" foods plus 2 bone broth snacks |

You have two mini-fast plans to choose from:

**Plan 1: Bone broth all day.** If you choose this plan, you can have up to 6 cups of broth during the day.

**Plan 2: Bone broth until 7 p.m., followed by a light snack or a Bone Broth Diet–approved shake.** If you sleep better when you have a small meal, you'll want to choose this option. (You'll find ideas for snacks in Chapter 4, and shake recipes in Chapter 11.)

Which plan you choose is totally up to you—and if you change your mind, you can switch at any time. So experiment and see which one works best for you.

You'll start a fast in the morning and end it 24 hours later. Basically, you'll skip a breakfast, lunch, and dinner, replacing them with broth (and with the 7 p.m. snack if you choose Plan 2).

On any day—fasting or not—you'll have "extras" you can reach for if you feel hungry. (I'll tell you about these later in the book.) So if you're worried about getting cravings, don't fret—I've totally got you covered!

By the way, while you're on your diet, I'd like you to avoid weighing yourself. I know it's hard—but constant weighing is misleading because your weight can go up or down due to hormone fluctuations, constipation, or even a little extra salt intake. So put that scale in the closet until your 21 days are up. You'll be able to tell when you're losing weight by noticing the way your clothes fit.

## HOW WILL YOUR NONFASTING DAYS WORK?

On these days, as I've noted, you'll eat three full meals, along with two bone broth snacks. And when I say meals, I mean *meals*—not tiny, sad little plates of food that depress you. You'll dine on entrees like Broiled Chipotle Flank Steak, Persian Lamb Shanks, Cuban Pulled Pork, and Baked Coconut Shrimp. You'll find yourself reaching for this cookbook *long* after your 21-day diet is over!

In Chapter 3, you'll discover all of the yummy foods you can choose from. In addition, I'll tell you exactly how to measure your portions so you can eat full, satisfying meals and still burn fat like mad.

## WHY DOES THE DIET LAST THREE WEEKS?

Actually, you can stay on this diet as long as you like. I have clients who've followed it for a year or more and lost hundreds of pounds. So think of 21 days as a *minimum*, not a maximum.

Are you wondering why I picked this number? I didn't select it arbitrarily. As a scientist and a researcher, I chose it for a good reason.

Think about it like this:

Your food makes your blood. Your blood makes your cells, and your cells make your organs. So if you give your body the right raw material in the form of anti-inflammatory foods, you will actually change the health of your organs. How powerful is that?

Now, here is something else I want you to think about. Your cells have different life spans:

- Red blood cells renew every month.
- Skin cells renew in 2 to 12 months.
- Bone cells renew in 2 to 6 years.
- Nerve cells renew in 2 to 7 years.
- Intestinal cells renew in 3 weeks.

That last number is the one I want you to think about right now. Remember how I explained why healing your gut is the biggest key to losing your extra pounds? Well, it takes your gut cells about three weeks to turn over.

I remember a patient telling me, "Dr. Kellyann, it's crazy, but I feel like my insides are getting cleaner or something." Well, they literally were. Her body was hitting the compost button and renewing itself every day. As a result, she was burning fat like crazy.

That's why sticking to this program for 21 days is so vital. That's when the magic happens.

## HEADS UP—BE READY FOR THE "CARB FLU!"

On this diet, you're going to flip your fat-burning switch from "off" to "on." That's because your cells will start burning fat instead of energy for fuel. As a result, you'll become a *fat-burning machine*.

This is exactly what you want to happen. However, it can result in temporary symptoms I call the *carb flu*. To be successful on this diet, you need to be prepared for this little unpleasantness. It may not happen to you, but if it does, don't let it derail your diet!

As I guide my patients on their transformations, this is one of the moments when I need them to stay strong. Make it past this stage, and I promise you—it gets easier. The biggest key is to recognize that the carb flu is a *good* thing, and it passes quickly.

Here's the deal. Right now, if you're eating a standard diet or even a so-called healthy diet that's high in carbs, your cells are lazy. You're constantly bathing them in sugar, so they don't need to work hard to get the fuel they need.

Burning fat takes more effort on their part, and at first, they're not going to like it. As a result, for three to seven days, you may feel "tired, cranky, wired, and weird." This is totally normal, and it's actually a great sign—it tells you that you're switching over to rapid fat-burning mode.

Here's a look at some of the symptoms you may experience during this brief transitional period.

# How You May Feel Early On

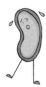   

| EXHAUSTED | "CARB FLU-ISH" | MOODY | ICKY |
|---|---|---|---|
| You might feel a bit low on energy, and that's completely normal. Be patient with yourself during this time, and try to keep your schedule light. If necessary, ease off the intensity of your workouts. Take a nap if you can, and aim to get to bed an hour earlier than usual so your body can rest and adapt. Also, try not to rely too much on caffeine to get you through afternoon slumps.<br><br>Right now, your body is beginning its transition from using sugar as fuel to burning fat—and that's what will turn you into a super-fat-burning machine. | It's not uncommon, especially if you've typically eaten a diet high in processed carbohydrates and fast food, to feel like you're getting a cold during this time. This is more evidence that your body is transitioning from using sugar as fuel to using fat.<br><br>So don't be alarmed if you feel tired or foggy-headed or get the sniffles. These are signs (and temporary ones!) that your diet is working the way it's supposed to. | Are you feeling short-tempered or moody for no reason? Actually, there *is* a reason: Your brain is throwing a hissy fit because it misses sugar, bread, and all the other foods you're not giving it.<br><br>Be patient. This will all pass in a few days, so don't give in to your cravings or your moodiness.<br><br>That moodiness, by the way, is related to your changing blood sugar levels. Eating real foods will eventually regulate your blood sugar and have you smiling again. | While you're making the transition to a super-fat-burning state, you may experience a few other odd symptoms. These can include digestive distress, allergies, and even a little acne.<br><br>These might get worse before they get better, but they will get better . . . soon! Remember that this is your body removing toxins and healing itself. It's just throwing a small temper tantrum while it does this. At the end of that tantrum, you'll be rewarded with a shrinking waistline, clearer skin, fewer wrinkles, glossier hair, and glowing health. |

The keys to getting through the carb flu are understanding why it's happening, remembering that it's temporary, and taking steps to make it easier on you.

Here are three tips for taming the carb flu:

- If you're hungry during this time, eat a handful of unsweetened coconut chips, a few pieces of avocado, or some olives with the salt rinsed off. This little "hit" of fat can make you feel better quicker.

- Journal every day. This will help you spot the signs of the carb flu and recognize when it's over.

- Diet with a friend if you can. You can give each other moral support when the carb flu strikes, and remind each other that it'll be over soon.

## A QUICK LOOK AT WHAT TO ANTICIPATE ON THE DIET

I've guided so many amazing weight-loss transformations that I've lost count—and in the process, I've learned what to expect, day by day. In fact, I've pretty much got it down to a science.

To prepare you for what's ahead, I've put together a quick road map for your 21 days. Of course, each of us is unique, so you may hit each milestone a little sooner or later than most people. However, here's what I predict as a general rule—along with the advice I give my patients at each stage.

### Day 1: The roller coaster

One minute, you're confident and in control. You're totally psyched. You're thinking, "This is gonna be a cinch."

The next minute, you're feeling overwhelmed and wondering, "OMG, what did I get myself into?"

MY ADVICE: Stay grounded and talk with supportive people.

### Days 2–7: The battleground

Right now, you're locked in hand-to-hand combat with the Sugar Demon and the carb flu. As a result, you feel cranky, tired, and maybe even a little sick.

MY ADVICE: Remember that this is *temporary*—and that you're breaking your sugar addiction and turning yourself into a fat-burning machine. So stay strong!

Also, remember my tip about easing your carb flu cravings with a little hit of fat. And if you're craving sugar, remember that the average craving lasts only three minutes. Play a game on your phone, call a friend, walk the dog, or answer some e-mails at work, and you'll outlast it. (A mug of bone broth will help stop sugar cravings, too.)

### Day 8: Whaaaat?

Your carb flu is gone, and you feel fantastic . . . until you put your clothes on. What the heck? They're *tighter*! You're stunned. You're thinking, "You *betrayed* me, Dr. Kellyann."

MY ADVICE: Relax! At this point, you're starting to change your microbiome—that ecosystem inside your gut. This can cause very temporary bloating, diarrhea, or constipation. It'll pass quickly—so please don't put out a hit on me.

### Days 9–11: Half-time doubts

The thrill of starting your diet is wearing off. You're tired of the broth. You're tired of cooking. You're missing your macaroni and cheese. And you're wondering, "Is this really worth it?" Based on my experience, this is the time when you're most likely to say, "I quit."

MY ADVICE: Remember why you started this diet. Think about your goals: a slimmer body, more beautiful skin, more energy, better health. You're halfway there, so think positive and resolve to stay the course.

### Days 12–15: Dream on!

Now you're feeling slimmer, younger, and stronger. Your doubts are gone, and you're aiming straight for the finish line. But at nighttime, a strange thing happens: You find yourself dreaming about gooey, sugary, carb-y foods. What's that all about?

MY ADVICE: I call these guilt-free doughnut dreams. Enjoy them—but don't give in to them. Your brain is trying to con you into going back to your old, fattening habits, but you don't need to listen.

### Days 16–18: Tiger blood

Oh, yeah, baby—now you're getting the picture. You're losing inches, you're feeling amazing, you have an insane amount of energy, and your skin looks years younger. In addition, you're experiencing that "tiger blood" I talked about earlier. It's like Valentine's Day every day.

MY ADVICE: Enjoy! And if you're still waiting for this amazing transition, be patient—it takes some people a little longer, but it'll happen.

### Days 19–20: This is so awesome—but now what?

As you head down the homestretch, you're on *fire*—looking fabulous, feeling fabulous, and ready to show the world your stuff. But after years of yo-yo dieting, you're worrying, "Will it last, or will I regain the weight just like I have in the past?"

MY ADVICE: Realize that you've now changed your relationship with food forever.

On the 80/20 Plan I'll talk about next, you'll be able to add "personal play" to your diet without gaining your weight back. From this point on, *you're in control.*

## Day 21: You did it!

Three short weeks ago, you asked yourself, "Can I really do this?" The answer is yes—and *you did it.* I'm so proud of you! You're slimmer, younger, sexier, healthier, and stronger, and you're thrilled with yourself for reaching your goal. Welcome to the brand-new you!

MY ADVICE: Celebrate! Buy new clothes. Buy new makeup. Get your hair done. Strut your stuff. Oh, and enjoy a glass of wine or a shot of potato vodka. You've earned it.

## A WORD ABOUT "OOPSIES"

Now that you know what to expect day by day, let's talk about one more thing: What happens if you slip up and have a "cheat" on one of these days?

Well, don't worry, because I'm not about to let you fail. (I told you I was the last-chance doctor, right?)

Here's the deal. If you "fall off the wagon," I don't want you to give up. I don't want you to think, "I'm a loser" or "I've messed up again." Instead, I want you to realize that you're *perfectly imperfect,* just like we all are, and simply start your 21-day countdown from the beginning again.

I want to emphasize this because I hate seeing people—especially women—beat themselves up over a diet "oopsie," as I call it. Unlike many other doctors, I have no interest in making you feel guilty if you give in to temptation. I'm not into guilt trips, because they just stress you out, and stress makes you even more likely to reach for a candy bar or a bag of chips.

Besides, feeling guilty is simply *illogical.* As I said earlier, sugar is addictive—and addiction can be hard to break. As a result, it may take you a few tries before you can walk away from those doughnuts and cupcakes.

It can also be hard to resist temptation if you take a big emotional hit—and I *totally* understand the urge to reach for ice cream or pizza if you're angry or sad. Believe me, I've been there myself. So again . . . if this happens, give yourself points for picking yourself up and starting again.

It is important to wind up spending 21 *consecutive* days on the diet, because that's what kicks your body into fat-burning mode. But you don't get only one shot at it. If it takes you a few tries to hit Day 21, that's perfectly fine.

So relax! Many of my most successful patients, including some who lost 50, 70, or even 100 pounds, had multiple "oopsies" before they made it through an entire 21 days. It didn't stop them from losing all of their extra weight. They just *restarted their 21-day clock again*—and that's what I want you to do.

## MY 80/20 MAINTENANCE PLAN: THE END OF YO-YO DIETING!

If you're a veteran of lots of diets, you may be thinking, "Sure, I can lose the weight. But won't I just gain it right back?" After all, that's what happens to nearly every dieter. In fact, people often gain back more weight than they lost.

But don't worry . . . I've got you covered here, too! (Hey, I'm not about to desert you *now*.)

Let's talk about what usually happens when you finish a diet. Normally, you go right back to eating the way you ate before. Why doesn't that work? *Because that's how you gained weight in the first place*. So that's not what I want you to do.

Instead, I want you to transition to my 80/20 Plan—or what I call the Bone Broth Diet Plus. On this plan, you'll follow the diet template for 80 percent of your meals and then eat what you want for the other 20 percent of your meals.

The fantastic thing about this plan is that it gives you 100 percent of the results with only 80 percent of the effort. For instance, you can order enchiladas and rice on Saturday night, or indulge in a pancake brunch on Sunday morning, without worrying about undoing your hard work. That's because you'll make so many investments in your "good health bank" over the rest of the week that you can get away with sprinkling on some occasional fairy dust.

On the 80/20 Plan, you'll have lots of room for that *personal play* I mentioned earlier. For instance, if you have autoimmune issues or you still want to lose a little more weight, try going 90/10. Or if you're happy with your weight and you're in great health, go ahead and use up your entire budget of cheats.

Here's a caution, however. As you reintroduce foods, I want you to pay close attention to how your body reacts to them. The results may surprise you. For instance, you may discover that your skin breaks out when you eat grains, that mashed potatoes make you feel bloated, or that cheese gives you a headache.

In particular, watch out if you reintroduce foods containing gluten. More than

80 percent of my patients have a bad reaction to foods containing gluten, and of all the foods you eliminated on the Bone Broth Diet, this is the one that's most likely to cause trouble for you. So really, really pay attention if you add gluten-containing foods back into your diet! To keep these foods in mind, remember the acronym BROWS. It stands for barley, rye, oats (which are okay *only* if they're specifically labeled as "gluten-free"), wheat, and spelt.

If you're really eager to add grains back into your diet, check out gluten-free grains like quinoa, millet, teff, amaranth, einkorn, emmer, and oatmeal that's specifically labeled as gluten-free. Also, if you're not familiar with grain-free flours like almond flour and coconut flour, give them a try—you'll be amazed at the fabulous desserts you can make. (Check out the desserts in Chapter 10 for ideas.)

Dairy is another food I want you to reintroduce cautiously, if at all. Dairy is a major cause of digestive problems, and many of my patients find that consuming milk or cheese leads to headaches, skin breakouts, or sinus problems.

These are the trickiest foods for most people, but you never know. So play Sherlock Holmes. Follow the clues your body sends, and get really, *really* smart about how the foods you eat affect your health, your mood, your skin, and your weight.

Now, let's talk a little about your sweet tooth. Once you're on the 80/20 Plan, you can have the occasional sweet treat. However, I recommend avoiding granulated white sugar because it's so bad for you. Instead, here are the sweeteners I recommend:

- Honey
- Blackstrap molasses
- Maple syrup
- Coconut sugar
- Date sugar (in small quantities)

Stevia is okay, too, although it's not at the top of my list. There's some evidence that stevia can increase insulin sensitivity, which is a good thing. But calorie-free sweeteners confuse your body, which is a bad thing. If you use lots of stevia because it's calorie-free, you're still training your body to expect too much sweetness, and you won't free yourself from the Sugar Demon. I turn to stevia only when other sweeteners can't do the job. If you do use it, buy pure stevia rather than brands that contain other additives.

## Play Detective!

If health problems like psoriasis or digestive upsets vanished while you were on the diet, I want you to be especially careful about adding foods back into your diet. In this situation, I recommend introducing a single new food at a time. Here's how to do it:

- Select a food to reintroduce. Eat enough of it that you'll be able to tell if you have a bad reaction, but don't overdo it.

- If you experience any of the following symptoms within 24 to 36 hours after adding a food, put it back on the "no" list. (You can retest that food later to see if your reaction was just a coincidence.)

  - Constipation, diarrhea, bloating, or gas
  - "Brain fog"
  - Headaches
  - Joint pain
  - Fatigue
  - Skin breakouts or rashes
  - Anxiety or depression

- Wait five days before introducing another food. This will make it much easier to determine how your body reacts to each food.

---

Next, here are a few words about alcohol. And those words are: It's fine now! (Yay!) If you add alcohol back into your diet, go for grain-free options like potato vodka (my favorite) or tequila. Wine is fine, too. If you like mixed drinks, skip the sugary mixers and go for muddled fruit, sparkling water, or a spritz of lemon instead. And, of course, limit yourself to one or two drinks when you're indulging.

Finally, let's talk about being beautifully imperfect—because we all are.

Here's the thing. It's easy to stay motivated on the 21-day diet, but it's a little harder to do what's right over the months and years that follow. So over time, you may slip up a little, and that 80/20 may become 70/30 or even 60/40. As a result, a few extra pounds and wrinkles may start to return.

If that's the case, don't kick yourself. Hey, you're only human! Simply go back on the original diet for 21 days, and then go right back on the 80/20 Plan. There's no need to ever worry again about your weight getting out of control—because you're in charge from this point on.

CHAPTER 3

# My Fabulous Fat-Burning Foods

BY THE TIME THEY reach my office, most of my patients have a long history of crazy diets. They've tried the cabbage diet. The grapefruit diet. The lemonade diet. The acai berry diet. The baby food diet. One of my clients almost got talked into doing the tapeworm diet, which involves swallowing . . . well, you can guess.

As a result, these patients have only one expectation: That like everyone else, I'm going to order them to eat weird, boring, or downright nasty stuff.

Luckily for them, they're absolutely *wrong*.

As you'll discover in this chapter, my diet is loaded with luscious, filling foods you're going to love. These foods are worthy of a spot on the menu at a gourmet restaurant. Serve them at dinner parties, and no one will ever guess that they're diet food. Share them with your family, and they'll ask for seconds.

All the while, these foods will be melting your fat off and blasting your wrinkles. These are the foods I use to help obese patients lose hundreds of pounds, to help Hollywood celebrities stay gorgeous and ageless, and to stay slim and wrinkle-free myself—and they're the foods that will turn you into a fat-burning machine.

In this chapter, I'll introduce you to these fabulous fat-burning foods. I think you'll be excited to see that you'll be feasting rather than starving on this diet. (If you're skeptical, go ahead and take a peek at the recipe sections. I'll wait right here for you.) And I think you're going to be happy when you discover that rather than eating microscopic portions, you'll fill your plate at each meal.

However . . .

Before we talk about the great foods you'll be enjoying, I want to talk about the flip side of the coin: the foods I want you to avoid on this diet. That's because I like to get the hard stuff out of the way first.

I'll admit right up front that there's a long list of "no" foods on my diet. However, you'll be swapping these foods out for so many fantastic foods that you aren't going to miss them much—especially when you see the pounds and inches vanish. (And you can reintroduce them during your 80/20 maintenance phase, if you choose.) So it's a temporary brush-off, and it's for a good cause: a slim, healthy new you!

## THE FOODS YOU'LL (TEMPORARILY) BID FAREWELL

There are several big food groups I'm asking you to avoid while you're on this diet. If they're favorites of yours, I know you'll feel a twinge when I tell you to toss them out.

However, I'm asking you to banish these foods for a good reason. Here's why they belong on the "no" list:

- **They flood your body with sugar, keeping it from burning fat for fuel.** To lose weight rapidly, you need to go into *ketosis*. This is the state in which your body begins burning ketone bodies—a type of fatty acid—for fuel. Many of my "no" foods are high in carbs, and you won't go into ketosis if you're giving your cells a steady supply of easy-to-burn sugar from these foods.
- **They cause chronic inflammation.** As I mentioned earlier, inflammatory foods pack on the weight—and our goal is to strip that weight off.
- **They damage your gut.** A glowing gut is the quickest route to fast weight loss and beautiful skin—and that means we need to cut out any food that makes your gut unhappy.

So trust me: If you're serious about transforming your body, these foods need to go. Give them to friends and family, donate them to food banks, or simply have someone store them for you until you're done with the diet. It's important to have them out of your house so you won't be tempted by them.

As I like to say, *be ruthless*. You have a big goal, so don't let anything stand in your way.

Now, here's a look at all of the foods on the "no" list. First I'll tell you what they are, and then I'll talk about why you need to eliminate them for now.

# FOODS YOU'LL ELIMINATE FOR THE NEXT THREE WEEKS

## Grains and Grain-Containing Foods

Barley

Breads

Cereal

Chips

Cookies

Cornstarch and other food starches

Crackers

Granola

Oats

Pasta

Quinoa

Rice

Rye

Spelt

Wheat

## Corn-Based Products

Corn

Popcorn

Products that contain corn oil (for instance, mayonnaise and salad dressings)

## Refined Processed Fats

Canola oil

Corn oil

Grapeseed oil

Margarine and vegetable shortening

Peanut oil

Safflower oil

Soybean oil

Sunflower oil

Vegetable oil

Any foods containing these fats

## Artificial Sweeteners

Acesulfame K

Aspartame

Saccharin

Stevia

Sucralose

Truvia

## Soy

Hoisin sauce

Soy hot dogs and other soy "meats"

Soy milk

Soy sauce

Teriyaki sauce

Tofu

## Dairy Products

Butter (except clarified butter—also called ghee; see page 64)

Cheese

Cream

Flavored creamers

Frozen yogurt

Half-and-half

Ice cream

Milk

Whey protein powder

Yogurt

## Commercial Condiments with Added Sugar or Artificial Ingredients

Barbecue sauce

Bottled salad dressings and marinades

Ketchup

Sweet-and-sour sauces

## Sugars

All sugars including honey, maple syrup, molasses, and jams and jellies

## Packaged Processed Foods

Including "healthy" processed foods in boxes or freezer containers, which often contain wheat, soy, sugars, or dairy

## Commercial Sauces, Soups, and Stews

These typically contain flour and artificial colors or flavors

## Canned Foods with Sugar, Soy, or Additives

Canned fruits packed in syrup

Canned tuna packed in soybean oil

Any other canned food with artificial ingredients or "mystery" ingredients

## Sodas, Fruit Juices, Sweetened Coffee/Tea, and Alcohol

Sugar-sweetened and artificially sweetened drinks

Wine, beer, and hard liquor

## Ice Pops and Frozen Fruit Bars with Sugar and/or Artificial Ingredients

## Processed Meats

Lunchmeats, bacon, and sausage containing gluten, nitrites, soy, or sweeteners

*Note: Lunchmeats, sausage, and bacon that don't contain these ingredients are fine.*

## White Potatoes

## Beans/Legumes

Beans

Lentils

Peanut butter

Peanuts

Peas

*Note: Green beans and sugar snap peas are fine.*

I believe that knowledge is power, so I want you to understand why these foods landed on my "no" list. Here's a look at why each one failed to make the cut.

## Sugar

Earlier, I mentioned that sugar is addictive. The more you eat, the more you want—and the more you want, the more weight you gain.

That's bad enough, but in addition, sugar is incredibly bad for you. In fact, it's even worse than you think.

I'm guessing you already know that sugar raises your blood sugar, wrecks your teeth, and puts pounds on you. But here's more bad news: It's also incredibly inflammatory. It elevates your levels of pro-inflammatory proteins called cytokines[1] and increases your body's production of substances called *advanced glycation end products*, or AGES.[2] AGES are *wildly* pro-inflammatory, and they make your skin wrinkle like crazy.

What's more, eating sugar raises your risk for developing cancer.[3] And if you eat a high-sugar diet, you dramatically increase your risk of dying from heart disease—even if the rest of your diet is healthy.[4]

In short, that sweet stuff is *very* bad news—so it's time to break the Sugar Demon's hold over you once and for all. It won't be easy, but once you're free, you'll never look back.

When you go sugar-free, make sure you avoid these "sneaky" forms of sugar as well:

| | |
|---|---|
| Agave nectar | Fruit juice concentrate |
| Barley malt syrup | Galactose |
| Cane crystals | Glucose |
| Corn sweetener | High-fructose corn syrup |
| Corn syrup | Invert sugar |
| Crystalline fructose | Lactose |
| Dehydrated cane juice | Maltodextrin |
| Dextrin | Maltose |
| Dextrose | Malt syrup |
| Disaccharide | Monosaccharide |
| Evaporated cane juice | Polysaccharide |
| Fructose | Ribose |

Rice syrup

Saccharose

Sorghum

Sorghum syrup

Sucrose

Treacle

Turbinado sugar

Xylose

## Artificial sweeteners

For years, diet "experts" told us to replace sugar with artificial sweeteners like aspartame, sucralose, and saccharin. But guess what: These sweeteners are as bad for you as sugar itself.

According to recent research, artificial sweeteners encourage the growth of certain bacteria that promote fat storage.[5] They also raise blood sugar,[6] putting you at increased risk for diabetes. And they feed your sugar cravings,[7] ensuring that the Sugar Demon keeps you in his clutches.

Besides that, artificial sweeteners are chemicals created in a laboratory. Your body isn't geared to handle them—and that means they're toxic to you.

One note here: Stevia is actually a *natural* sweetener that comes from a plant and is okay in small doses on the 80/20 Plan (see Chapter 2). However, for now, I want you to avoid stevia as well. Sweet foods have too much power over your life right now, and I want you to take that power back.

## Grains

This one tends to make people flip out. "But grains are *good* for me!" they tell me. Well, no . . . they aren't.

Evolutionarily speaking, grains are a very new food in our diet—and that means we aren't designed to eat them. What's more, wheat and other popular grains are now so genetically modified that they bear little resemblance to the grains we ate even a few decades ago. As a result, our bodies don't handle them well, leading to a leaky gut and inflammation.[8]

In addition to being pro-inflammatory, grains make your blood sugar soar. To your body, there's really no difference between the sugar in a bowl of pasta and the sugar in a cookie—and either one will lead to spiking blood glucose, rising insulin levels, and more fat around your belly.

So I want you to cross all grains off your list for now. It's especially crucial to avoid gluten, which can wreak havoc on your gut. Here are some sneaky ingredients that indicate that a food definitely or possibly contains gluten:

| | |
|---|---|
| Artificial flavoring | Modified food starch |
| Bleached flour | Natural flavoring |
| Caramel color | Seasonings |
| Dextrin | Vegetable protein |
| Hydrolyzed plant protein (HPP) | Vegetable starch |
| Hydrolyzed wheat protein | Wheat germ oil |
| Hydrolyzed wheat starch | Wheat grass |
| Malt | Wheat protein |
| Maltodextrin | Wheat starch |

Corn is a grain, too, so avoid anything containing it. Watch out for these sneaky ingredients, which possibly or definitely indicate the presence of corn:

| | |
|---|---|
| Artificial flavoring | Maltodextrin |
| Corn alcohol | Mazena |
| Corn flour | Modified gum starch |
| Cornmeal | MSG |
| Corn oil | Natural flavorings |
| Cornstarch | Sorbitol |
| Corn sweetener | Vegetable gum |
| Corn syrup solids | Vegetable protein |
| Dextrin | Vegetable starch |
| Dextrose | Xanthan gum |
| Food starch | Xylitol |
| High-fructose corn syrup | |

## Dairy

One thing that surprises me when I tell people about the "no" foods on this diet is the number of people who say, "I can't do it. I can give up cookies and sodas and french fries, but there's no way I can drink my coffee without milk."

To me, it's amazing that this seemingly tiny sacrifice is a potential deal breaker. But it actually makes sense, because dairy—like sugar—is addictive.[9] Dairy products contain opioid peptides similar to the endorphins your body manufactures to make you feel good. Over time, you've come to enjoy that little "hit of happiness," so you're actually going to suffer a tiny bit of withdrawal when you say goodbye to dairy products.

So why should you cut out dairy when you're on my diet? Because a large majority of people don't handle dairy well—and most of them don't realize it until they give it up. That's when their headaches, bloating, gas, and skin breakouts clear up.

Chances are, you too have symptoms that stem from dairy—and you'll never know unless you go "cold turkey" for a little while. So trust me: It's worth drinking your coffee black (or with coconut milk) for a few weeks. You can add dairy right back into your diet when you reach the 80/20 Plan, if you choose.

## Soy

Do your doctors tell you to eat lots of soy because it's good for you? I strongly disagree—and for good reason. Here's the rap sheet on this so-called health food:

- Soy puts you at risk for an underactive thyroid, which can make you fat and sluggish. It also suppresses your uptake of iodine, a nutrient crucial for healthy thyroid function, and promotes thyroid autoimmunity.[10]

- Soy contains phytoestrogens that alter your hormone levels. Women who drink the equivalent of 2 cups of soy milk per day get the estrogenic equivalent of one birth control pill.[11] This can cause *estrogen dominance*, throwing your hormones out of whack and making you gain weight.

- Soy "Frankenfoods," like burgers, hot dogs, and sausage, are often heavily processed and contain MSG—a toxin that excessively stimulates your cells. Many soy products also contain the toxic chemicals lysinoalanine and nitrosamines, which damage your cells, leading to inflammation.

By the way, it's not true that a healthy Asian diet centers around soy. In reality, there's very little soy in traditional Asian diets, and it's usually fermented and unprocessed, unlike the soy that manufacturers use in Western countries.

When you give soy the boot for the next 21 days, be sure to eliminate all of these soy-containing foods as well:

| | |
|---|---|
| Hydrolyzed plant protein (HPP) | Stabilizer |
| Hydrolyzed soy protein | Tamari |
| Hydrolyzed vegetable protein (HVP) | Tempeh |
| Miso natural flavoring | Textured soy flour (TSF) |
| Soy albumin | Textured soy protein (TSP) |
| Soy fiber | Textured vegetable protein (TVP) |
| Soy flour | Tofu vegetable broth |
| Soy lecithin | Vegetable gum |
| Soy protein | Vegetable starch |
| Soy sauce | |

## Industrial seed oils

Many so-called health experts will tell you that seed oils like corn, soybean, sunflower, and canola oil are good for you. However, these oils are heavily processed and frequently rancid even at the time you buy them.

Worse yet, most seed oils have an unhealthy ratio of omega-6 to omega-3 fatty acids. They're high in omega-6s, which are pro-inflammatory, and low in anti-inflammatory omega-3s. Remember that the quickest way to lose weight is to reduce inflammation—so we don't want anything in your diet that's going to *increase* that inflammation instead.

You may be surprised to see canola oil on my "no" list, because it's touted as a health food (and because its ratio of omega-3 to omega-6 is better than for other seed oils). But in reality, canola oil isn't even *close* to healthy. If you aren't familiar with the origins of canola oil, it's made from a plant called rapeseed that had to be genetically modified for human use because of its extreme toxicity. Even now, canola oil undergoes so much refining, bleaching, deodorizing, and "degumming" that it's hardly a food at all. Trust me: There are better ways to get your omega-3s!

## Legumes and potatoes

These two foods are on the "no" list because they're high in carbohydrates that turn straight into sugar, and you want your cells to be burning fat instead. Beans are also hard to digest—that's why they're nicknamed the "musical fruit"—and you don't want to stress your gut while you're working hard to heal it. So cross them off your list for now.

During your 80/20 maintenance phase, you may find that you can handle beans without any problems. An occasional potato will be just fine then, too. But for now, avoid these foods.

## Artificial ingredients

Imagine that it's morning, and I offer to make breakfast for you. Wow—that's nice of me, right? But to your surprise, I don't hand you a plate of eggs, fruit, or bacon. Instead, I hand you dozens of chemicals mixed together in a test tube.

Now, suppose I tell you that these chemicals have no nutritional value at all. Worse yet, many of them may be bad for you. They may increase your inflammation, put you at higher risk for diabetes, or even make you more vulnerable to cancer.

Would you drink what's in that test tube? I'm pretty confident that you wouldn't. But you're doing the equivalent every day if you eat a diet that's high in fake colors, flavorings, thickeners, and fillers. According to the Environmental Working Group, there are more than 10,000 additives allowed in processed food.[12]

Manufacturers like to say that these chemicals are safe, but I don't buy into that myth. First of all, *any* artificial substance you put in your body confuses your cells because they're not engineered to handle it—and this confusion messes with your metabolism, your hormone levels, and your immune system. Second, there's strong evidence that many of these chemicals are indeed very dangerous. For instance, here are some of the "generally recognized as safe" chemicals in processed foods:

- Potassium bromate, added to foods like breads and crackers, is listed as a known carcinogen by the state of California.[13]
- Propyl paraben can spur the growth of breast cancer cells.[14]

- BHA, used as a preservative, is an endocrine disruptor that alters your hormones, and the U.S. National Toxicology Program says it is "reasonably anticipated to be a human carcinogen."[15]

And the story gets even worse when you realize that a single processed food can contain half a dozen or more artificial chemicals. Scientists have *no* idea what happens when you start mixing these chemicals together. In effect, they're using you as a human guinea pig.

This is why I want you to avoid any foods with additives during your 21-day diet (and preferably after that). I want you to put only those foods in your body that optimize its function—not foods that slow down your metabolism, unbalance your hormones, or damage your cells.

## Alcohol

You're thinking about walking away right now, aren't you? And honestly, I don't blame you. I love a shot of potato vodka or a glass of wine after a hard day, so I know it's asking a lot of you to go without your favorite adult beverage.

Unfortunately, alcohol can damage your gut, making it leaky—and for this diet to succeed, you need your gut to be super healthy. In addition, alcohol can weaken your resolve, making it easier for you to stray from your diet. It also ages your skin, and right now we want to *de-age* it instead.

So hand your booze off to a friend—someone you can trust not to drink it!—and then collect it at the end of Day 21 so you can have a celebration toast. (For suggestions on preferred alcoholic drinks and mixers, see page 23.)

## THE GLORIOUS FOODS YOU'LL EAT ON MY DIET

Whew. Okay, that's all the hard stuff. Now let's get to the good stuff!

As I've said, you're going to eat *awesome* food on this diet. While you may pine temporarily for cheese puffs and French toast, I'm going to give you so many luscious alternatives that you'll quickly start looking forward to meals. And in addition to tasting good, these foods will make you feel good about yourself, because they'll be slimming, repairing, and de-aging your body from head to toe.

Here's a list of my "yes" foods. Skim through it, and then I'll tell you what these foods will do for you.

# YOUR FAT-BURNING BONE BROTH DIET "YES" FOODS

## Meats

Beef

Chicken

Lamb

Turkey

Wild boar

*Note: Buy pastured meat and free-range poultry if you can afford them. Avoid pork unless you can find pastured pork.*

## Bone Broth

Beef, lamb, chicken, turkey, or fish broth

## Fish

Fresh or canned. Buy wild-caught fish if possible, and make sure canned fish is packed in water or olive oil.

## Eggs

Buy organic/free range if possible.

## Organ Meats

Look for organic liver.

## Nitrite- and Gluten-Free Deli Meats, Bacon, and Sausages

*Note: Read labels carefully and make sure you're not getting any sugars or artificial ingredients.*

## Vegetables

Acorn squash

Artichokes

Arugula

Asparagus

Beets

Bell peppers

Bok choy

Broccoli

Broccoli rabe

Brussels sprouts

Butternut squash

Carrots

Cauliflower

Celery

Celery root

Chile peppers

Cilantro

Cucumber

Eggplant

Garlic

Green beans

Green cabbage

Green onions

Greens (beet, collard, mustard, and turnip greens)

Jalapeño chile peppers

Jicama

*(continued)*

Kale

Kohlrabi

Leeks

Lettuce

Mushrooms

Napa cabbage

Onions

Parsnips

Plantains

Pumpkin

Radicchio

Radishes

Red cabbage

Rutabaga

Seaweed

Snap peas

Snow peas

Spaghetti squash

Spinach

Sprouts

Summer squash

Sweet potatoes and yams

Swiss chard

Tomatoes (including canned or sun-dried tomatoes)

Turnips

Watercress

Yucca

Zucchini

*Notes: Eat starchy vegetables like sweet potatoes, winter squash, and pumpkin sparingly. Add them to a meal only if you need extra fuel after a workout, or you're feeling weak and tired and you know it isn't the carb flu.*

*Buy organic veggies if possible.*

*Corn is not on this list and is not Bone Broth Diet-approved.*

## Fruits

Apples

Applesauce, unsweetened

Apricots

Bananas

Blackberries

Blueberries

Cantaloupe

Cherries

Dates

Figs

Grapefruit

Grapes

Guava

Honeydew melon

Kiwifruit

Lemons

Limes

Mandarin oranges

Mangoes

Nectarines

Oranges

Papayas

Peaches

Pears

Pineapple

Plums

Pomegranates

Raspberries

Rhubarb

Strawberries

Tangerines

Ugli fruit

Watermelon

*Note: Buy organic if possible; also, empha-size berries, which are lower in sugar than most fruits. Avoid dried fruits, fruit juices, and smoothies—other than smoothies that contain only foods allowed on the diet.*

## Healthy Fats

Avocado oil

Avocados

Coconut

Coconut milk

Coconut oil

Ghee (clarified butter—see page 64)

Nuts

Olive oil

Olives

Tallow

## Healthy Meal-Replacement Shakes

*These shakes must have protein only from one of the Dr. Kellyann–approved sources.*

Collagen protein

Egg protein

Hydro beef protein

Pea protein (not optimal but okay)

*Note: To read the discussion "Beef Protein vs. Whey Protein," go to the Resources page on my Web site, bonebrothdietbook.com/resources.*

## Fermented Foods

Coconut kefir

Kimchi

Pickles, unpasteurized and refrigerated

Sauerkraut

## Condiments

Cocoa powder, unsweetened

Coconut aminos (to replace soy sauce)

Fish sauce

Hot sauce, gluten-free

Mustard, gluten-free

Pepper

Pickles, unsweetened and sulfite-free

Salsa

Salt, Celtic or pink Himalayan (instead of regular table salt)

Spices

Vinegar

*Note: While regular table salt contains iodine, it also contains additives you don't want. To get a good supply of iodine, be sure to include sea vegetables (like SeaSnax) and fish in your diet.*

### Flours and Thickeners

Almond flour

Arrowroot powder

Coconut flour

### Beverages

Coffee

Mineral water

Sparkling water

Tea

*Note: Try not to overdo caffeinated coffee or tea if you're experiencing the carb flu—instead, add a little extra fat to your diet to ease your symptoms.*

For shopping guides, specific brands, and recommendations, visit my Resources page on bonebrothdietbook.com/resources.

Why have I chosen these foods? Here are the reasons they made it over my *very* high bar.

- They're overflowing with nutrients that heal your gut, promote the formation of wrinkle-smoothing collagen in your skin, and optimize your hormones.

- They're loaded with powerful fat-burners like conjugated linoleic acid, choline, and lauric acid.

- Some are potent prebiotics (which create a healthy "soil" for your gut bugs) or probiotics (which repopulate your gut with these bugs).

- Some ramp up your liver's detoxification pathways, cleansing your body.

- Many are inflammation fighters, melting away pounds—especially the pounds around your belly.

- All of them are low in carbohydrates (except for some starchy veggies you'll eat only when you need them). As a result, they put your body into ketosis, flipping your fat-burning switch to "on" and making your extra weight disappear.

Each food on my list is a nutritional powerhouse. Better yet, when you combine them, the effects are synergistic. That's because nutrients power each other up. (For instance, eating healthy fats helps your body absorb crucial nutrients like the lycopene in tomatoes and the lutein in spinach.)

# Can You Modify the Bone Broth Diet If You're a Vegetarian? You Bet!

Here's one question I hear all the time: "Can I do this diet if I'm a vegetarian, a pescatarian, or a vegan?" The answer is a resounding *yes*.

While proteins like beef, chicken, and fish are part of the Bone Broth Diet, I'm all about personal play. I've altered this diet quite a few times to make it work for patients who choose to avoid many or all animal products, and it still works like magic.

Here's how to switch things up if you want to go meat-free:

- Let's start with the broth. Obviously, you can't make bone broth without bones! But that's fine, because you can substitute a rich vegetable broth. If you're a pescatarian—that is, you eat fish—you can also make a lovely, subtle broth out of fish bones.

- If you're a vegetarian, make eggs a big part of your diet. (Science has shown that eating eggs *isn't* bad for your cholesterol; for more on this, see page 88.) In addition, you can stretch the basic diet template to include beans and lentils, edamame, full-fat grass-fed kefir and yogurt, natto, and tempeh. High-quality vegetarian protein mixes, such as hemp or pea protein, are also acceptable as part of the vegetarian protocol.

- Avoid soy burgers, tofu hot dogs, and other processed soy foods. As I discussed earlier, these are *loaded* with unhealthy ingredients.

It may take a little longer to lose your extra pounds when you substitute beans, lentils, and other high-carb foods for animal proteins—but you'll still see amazing results. And even without the collagen building blocks from bone broth, you'll blast your wrinkles with skin-smoothing foods like coconut and avocado. In just 21 days, you'll be slimmer, look younger, and feel more energetic, without having to compromise on your dietary principles.

So join the Bone Broth Revolution—we're happy to have you on board!

---

This is why you're not going to skimp on my diet. You're going to load your plate with fat-burning, wrinkle-erasing, de-aging foods that will work together to transform your body.

## PORTION CONTROL: A BIG KEY TO SUCCESS

I'm not one of those doctors who want you to measure out your food with a scale or count calories on a calculator. That takes all the joy out of eating—and as an Italian girl, I want eating to be *fun*! I also know that reducing eating to an exercise in weighing and counting doesn't work, because it's frustrating and people just quit doing it.

Besides, all that work is simply *unnecessary*. And by now, you know that I don't believe in asking you to do anything that's unnecessary!

Choosing portions doesn't require scales, calculators, or point systems. This is a skill you were born with, and it won't take you long to relearn it. But first, let's talk about why you *unlearned* it.

As an infant, you knew when you'd eaten enough. But over time, you've been "untrained" by restaurants. As a result, it's all too easy to accept the idea that a half-pound burger with two cups of fries is a single serving—and that a tiny half-cup of broccoli or green beans is also a serving.

Luckily, it's pretty easy to relearn the art of natural portion control. Here's a simple chart that tells you how to eyeball your food accurately and make sure you aren't getting too much or too little. And on the page that follows, you'll find an At-a-Glance Meal Plan that shows you how to calculate your servings at each meal.

For more information, check out my Bone Broth Diet Quick Plate on my Resources page at bonebrothdietbook.com/resources.

# Easy Tips for Portion Control
## *A Perfect Plate*

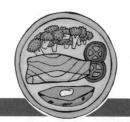

### PROTEIN PORTIONS

A serving of meat, fish, or poultry should be about the size and thickness of your palm. A serving of eggs is as many whole eggs as you can hold in your hand (that's about 2 or 3 for women and 3 or 4 for men). A serving of egg whites alone is double the serving for whole eggs. Each meal should include a serving of protein.

### NONSTARCHY VEGETABLE PORTIONS

A serving of these vegetables should be at least the size of a softball. You can't eat too many of them, so fill your plate with at least 2 or 3 softballs' worth.

### STARCHY VEGETABLE PORTIONS

A serving of starchy vegetables (such as sweet potato, jicama, kohlrabi, or winter squash) should be about the size of a baseball for women and the size of a softball for men. *Note:* Eat starchy vegetables only if you're recovering from a workout or you're feeling weak and tired and you know it's not the carb flu.

### FRUIT PORTIONS

A serving of fruit is half an individual piece (half an apple, half an orange) or a tennis-ball-size serving of berries, grapes, or tropical fruits (about ½ cup). That's a closed fistful, or about ½ cup, if they're diced. Eat no more than 2 servings of fruit per day, and break them up across meals and snacks to distribute your sugar intake.

### FAT PORTIONS

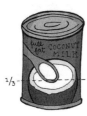

A serving of liquid fat should be about the size of a Ping-Pong ball, a typical bouncy ball, or 1 to 2 thumb-size portions (that's about 1 tablespoon).

A serving of nuts, seeds, coconut flakes, or olives is about 1 closed handful.

A serving of avocado is one-quarter to one-half an avocado.

A serving of coconut milk is one-third to one-half the can.

Each meal should include 1 or 2 servings of fat.

# At-a-Glance
## *Meal Plan*

| | BREAKFAST | LUNCH | DINNER | SNACK |
|---|---|---|---|---|
| **Day 1** | 1 portion protein<br>1 portion fat<br>1 portion fruit | 1 portion protein<br>2 portions vegetables<br>1 portion fat | 1 portion protein<br>2 portions vegetables<br>1 portion fat | Bone broth* |
| **Day 2** | Sip on bone broth. May also drink:<br>Coffee (black only)/tea<br>Water | Sip on bone broth. May also drink:<br>Coffee (black only)/tea<br>Water | Sip on bone broth. May also drink:<br>Coffee (black only)/tea<br>Water | Bone broth if you're doing Plan 1, or 7 p.m. snack or approved shake if you're doing Plan 2 |
| **Day 3** | 1 portion protein<br>1 portion fat<br>1 portion fruit | 1 portion protein<br>2 portions vegetables<br>1 portion fat | 1 portion protein<br>2 portions vegetables<br>1 portion fat | Bone broth* |
| **Day 4** | 1 portion protein<br>1 portion fat<br>1 portion fruit | 1 portion protein<br>2 portions vegetables<br>1 portion fat | 1 portion protein<br>2 portions vegetables<br>1 portion fat | Bone broth* |
| **Day 5** | Sip on bone broth. May also drink:<br>Coffee (black only)/tea<br>Water | Sip on bone broth. May also drink:<br>Coffee (black only)/tea<br>Water | Sip on bone broth. May also drink:<br>Coffee (black only)/tea<br>Water | Bone broth if you're doing Plan 1, or 7 p.m. snack or approved shake if you're doing Plan 2 |
| **Day 6** | 1 portion protein<br>1 portion fat<br>1 portion fruit | 1 portion protein<br>2 portions vegetables<br>1 portion fat | 1 portion protein<br>2 portions vegetables<br>1 portion fat | Bone broth* |
| **Day 7** | 1 portion protein<br>1 portion fat<br>1 portion fruit | 1 portion protein<br>2 portions vegetables<br>1 portion fat | 1 portion protein<br>2 portions vegetables<br>1 portion fat | Bone broth* |

*When you're feeling tired or weak or need energy, up to 2 mugs of bone broth are allowed per day for a snack.

## AVOIDING PITFALLS

As a weight-loss transformation expert, I know all the tricks for taking weight off successfully—and I also know all the pitfalls that can trip you up. Here's a look at how to troubleshoot two problems that might pop up during your diet.

### Are you hungry?

I *never* want you to feel like you're starving on this diet. So if you feel hungry, I want you to take action immediately!

Here are the two most common reasons why you might feel hungry, along with solutions for each one:

- During the carb flu, you might experience some food cravings. If this happens, what your body really needs is a little extra fat. So reach for those healthy fats I talked about earlier—some pieces of avocado, a handful of unsweetened coconut chips, or some olives rinsed of salt.

- At other times during your diet, you may need more food because you've burned off a lot of energy. The solution here is to add a serving of starchy "energy" vegetables to your next meal—for instance, half a sweet potato or some beets.

During your diet, always make sure you have a little stash of these "rescue" foods both at home and at work. I like to keep carrot sticks and jicama slices on hand all the time in case I need an energy boost.

Also, make sure you drink plenty of water. Often when people think they're hungry, they're actually thirsty. I recommend starting your morning with a glass of water spritzed with a little lemon juice, and drinking water every few hours throughout the day.

## Is your weight loss slower than you'd like?

Typically, people lose weight rapidly on my diet once they get past the carb flu stage and enter ketosis. Every once in a while, however, the pounds don't seem to be melting away. If this happens to you, here are my secrets for jump-starting your weight loss:

- **Eat less fruit.** Fruit is good for you, but it contains more natural sugar than the other foods on my diet—and that can keep your insulin levels too high. Be sure to limit yourself to a closed handful of berries or chopped fruit, or half of a larger piece of fruit like a pear.

- **Eat fewer nuts.** Again, stick to a closed handful. Nuts are a great food, but it's easy to overindulge if you aren't paying attention.

- **Make sure all "no" foods are out of your house.** Having them around makes it too easy to fall for temptation.

- **Make sure you're measuring your fats right.** Either too little or too much fat can slow your weight loss.

- **Double-check your other portions.** Be careful not to overdo it on protein—and not to *under*do it on nonstarchy vegetables.

- **Give up that last vice. Yeah, you know the one I'm talking about.** Maybe it's a nightly glass of wine or a teaspoon of sugar in your coffee. Whatever it is, kiss it goodbye for now. This is a no-compromises diet, so be strong.

Also, be aware that if you have a severely damaged gut due to frequent antibiotic use or other causes, it may take longer to get that glowing gut you need for rapid weight loss. Just be patient and keep doing all the right things, and the magic will happen!

## CHAPTER 4

# Making the Bone Broth Diet Super Easy

**IF YOU'RE ACCUSTOMED TO** microwaved meals or take-out food, I know that you may be feeling a little intimidated by the idea of eating fresh, healthy foods at every meal. But relax—I have simple solutions for you!

First, I'm going to show you how to make food prep easy and efficient on the Bone Broth Diet. You'll minimize your kitchen time, fill your fridge and freezer with beautiful food, and never fall prey to what I call the six o'clock panic. That's when you're exhausted and hungry, you need something to eat *now*, and you're tempted to dial up the pizza place and kiss your diet goodbye.

Instead, you're going to be prepared. You're going to always, always have ready-to-eat "yes" foods at your fingertips. The secret to this, as you'll learn in this chapter, is a trick called *batch cooking*.

Batch cooking simply means setting aside one morning or afternoon each week to prepare meals ahead of time. For instance, you can roast two chickens, boil a dozen eggs, prep some veggies, and cook a big pot of chili. Then you'll simply freeze or refrigerate your bounty in single-serving containers, and voilà! You're set for days.

I'll also tell you how to make sure you're stocked up for your 7 p.m. snack, if you choose this option for your mini-fasting days. Plus, I'll give you a complete shopping list so you can have every ingredient for my recipes on hand—and I'll give you advice for shopping wisely and resisting temptation at the grocery store.

Finally, I'm going to give you plenty of ideas for no-cook meals. While I'm assuming that you like to cook—after all, you're reading a cookbook!—you may also enjoy the occasional grab-and-go meal from the grocery store. When you combine some quick store-bought meals with batch-cooked feasts, you'll never need to worry about what's for breakfast, lunch, or dinner.

## MY BEST TIPS FOR BATCH COOKING

I've been batch cooking for years, and it's a warm and cozy habit for me. I look forward to spending a Saturday morning or Sunday afternoon cooking with my kids, because it's a great way for us to build memories. And you know what? My boys are becoming better cooks than I am!

Of course, my sons and I also have lots of other things to do on weekends—so over the years, I've learned how to make batch cooking go faster with the help of a few simple tricks. Here are my favorites.

### Before you start. . . .

The first thing you'll want to do, even before you select recipes to batch cook, is to make sure you have plenty of single-serving containers (or family-size containers, if you're cooking for more than one). I prefer glass because it's toxin-free, but if you have plastic, that's okay, too.

You can use Mason jars, but make sure you cool them completely before freezing them. Also—and this is critical—leave an inch or more of space at the top to allow the food to expand when you freeze it.

Stock up on different sizes of freezer bags as well. If you have a food sealer, better yet—but regular bags will do fine, too.

In addition, it's helpful to have at least a couple of timers. This way, you can time different cooking projects simultaneously. It's a good idea to set a note by each timer, reminding you of which dish it's timing.

If you have a little extra cash, buy a few gadgets that will make batch cooking easier. I love spiralizers, which quickly turn zucchini or other veggies into noodles. In addition, an extra set of measuring cups and spoons will come in handy.

Now, pick out the recipes you want to make. You can choose any recipes you like, or follow my handy 3-Week Meal Plan in this chapter. If you create your own plan, look for recipes that share ingredients like chopped onions, chopped bell peppers, minced garlic, or sliced mushrooms. That way, you'll minimize your work.

And this is critical: Plan on making at least one week's worth of bone broth *before* you start your diet! Bone broth is fun and easy to make, and you can squeeze it into any batch cooking project.

## As you cook. . . .

It's smart to set out all of your ingredients at the beginning of your batch cooking project. (Professional chefs call this *mise en place*.) That way, you'll know you have everything on hand and won't need to make a mad dash to the grocery store!

Aim to complete four or five cooking projects, but don't overload yourself. Pick a couple of big projects—for instance, a double batch of soup or chili and a pot roast—and then plan on a few smaller ones, like hard-cooked eggs and a double batch of cauliflower rice (which cooks in minutes).

Clean up as you go. This guarantees that you'll always have clean tools, bowls, and pans ready to grab for the next project.

Cut up celery, carrots, radishes, and onions, and store them in water in individual containers. That way, they'll stay crunchy. Wash tomatoes and cucumbers so they're ready to grab, and spin any greens that aren't prewashed. If you have time, lightly steam some broccoli, carrots, green beans, or Brussels sprouts, or roast some root vegetables like carrots, beets, and turnips.

## When you're finished. . . .

Be sure to label everything before you store it. That way, you'll know what you have at a glance. Also, date each container.

To freeze meatballs, first place them on a baking sheet and prefreeze them for about 30 minutes. When they're hard, you can put them in freezer bags without flattening them.

## 3 WEEKS OF MEAL PLANS

In addition to making your meals fun, I want your meal planning to be as easy as possible. That's because I know that like me, you already have way too much to do every day.

So to simplify things for you, I've developed three weeks of complete meal plans that allow you to cut down on cooking time and make great use of your leftovers. Note that each week includes five days of meals, since you'll be doing bone broth mini-fasts on the other two days.

# Meal Plan
## Week 1

| | BREAKFAST | LUNCH | DINNER |
|---|---|---|---|
| **Day 1** | Ham and Eggs to Go (page 91)<br>Portions: 1 protein, ½ fat, 1 vegetable<br>(serve leftovers for Day 3 breakfast)<br><br>Handful of berries<br>Portion: 1 fruit | Asian Chicken Hash (page 108)<br>Portions: 1 protein, ¼ fat, 1 vegetable<br>(serve leftovers for Day 4 lunch)<br><br>Grilled Garden Salad with Green Goddess Dressing (page 164)<br>Portions: 1 fat, 2 vegetable<br>(serve leftovers for Day 2 lunch) | Grilled Salmon with Spiced Blueberry Sauce (page 154)<br>Portions: 1 protein, 1 fat, ½ fruit<br>(serve leftovers for Day 3 lunch)<br><br>Garden salad with any Bone Broth Diet salad dressing<br>Portions: ½ fat, 1 vegetable |
| **Day 2** | Pico de Gallo Eggs (page 92)<br>Portions: 1 protein, ½ fat<br>(serve leftovers for Day 4 breakfast)<br><br>Handful of berries<br>Portion: 1 fruit | Turkey Kale Meatballs with Zucchini Noodles and Salsa Cruda (page 112)<br>Portions: 1 protein, ½ fat, 2 vegetable<br>(serve leftovers for Day 4 dinner)<br><br>Grilled Garden Salad with Green Goddess Dressing<br>(leftovers from Day 1 lunch)<br>Portions: 1 fat, 2 vegetable | Cave Man or Woman Burgers (page 124)<br>Portions: 1 protein, ½ fat, 1 vegetable<br>(serve leftovers for Day 5 dinner)<br><br>Sizzling Sesame Scallions (page 173)<br>Portions: ½ fat, ¼ vegetable<br>(serve leftovers for Day 4 lunch) |
| **Day 3** | Ham and Eggs to Go<br>(leftovers from Day 1 breakfast)<br>Portions: 1 protein, ½ fat, 1 vegetable<br><br>Handful of berries<br>Portion: 1 fruit | Grilled Salmon with Spiced Blueberry Sauce<br>(leftovers from Day 1 dinner)<br>Portions: 1 protein, 1 fat, ½ fruit<br><br>Garden salad with any Bone Broth Diet salad dressing<br>Portions: ½ fat, 1 vegetable | Colorful Beef Stir-Fry (page 122)<br>Portions: 1 protein, 1 fat, 1 vegetable<br>(serve leftovers for Day 5 lunch) |
| **Day 4** | Pico de Gallo Eggs<br>(leftovers from Day 2 breakfast)<br>Portions: 1 protein, ½ fat<br><br>Handful of berries<br>Portion: 1 fruit | Asian Chicken Hash<br>(leftovers from Day 1 lunch)<br>Portions: 1 protein, ¼ fat, 1 vegetable<br><br>Sizzling Sesame Scallions<br>(leftovers from Day 2 dinner)<br>Portions: ½ fat, ¼ vegetable | Turkey Kale Meatballs with Zucchini Noodles and Salsa Cruda<br>(leftovers from Day 2 lunch)<br>Portions: 1 protein, ½ fat, 2 vegetable |
| **Day 5** | Sweet Potato Sausage Hash (page 94)<br>Portions: 1 protein, ¼ fat, ½ vegetable, 1 starchy vegetable<br><br>Handful of berries<br>Portion: 1 fruit | Colorful Beef Stir-Fry<br>(leftovers from Day 3 dinner)<br>Portions: 1 protein, 1 fat, 1 vegetable | Cave Man or Woman Burgers<br>(leftovers from Day 2 dinner)<br>Portions: 1 protein, ½ fat, 1 vegetable<br><br>Sriracha-Glazed Turnips (page 172)<br>Portions: ¼ fat, 1 starchy vegetable |

# Meal Plan
## Week 2

| | BREAKFAST | LUNCH | DINNER |
|---|---|---|---|
| **Day 1** | Salmon Stacks (page 93)<br>Portions: 1 protein, 1 fat<br>(serve leftovers for Day 3 breakfast)<br><br>Handful of berries<br>Portion: 1 fruit | Spicy Braised Chicken Thighs with Fried Capers (page 119)<br>Portions: 1 protein, 1 fat, 1 vegetable<br>(serve leftovers for Day 4 lunch)<br><br>Cauliflower Fried Rice (page 168)<br>Portions: ¼ protein, ¼ fat, 1 vegetable<br>(serve leftovers for Day 2 lunch) | Stuffed Peppers (page 127)<br>Portions: 1 protein, ½ fat, 2 vegetable<br>(serve leftovers for Day 3 lunch)<br><br>Garden salad with any Bone Broth Diet salad dressing<br>Portions: ½ fat, 1 vegetable |
| **Day 2** | Soft-Cooked Eggs with Yucca "Soldiers" (page 95)<br>Portions: ½ protein, ¼ fat, 1 starchy vegetable<br>(serve leftovers for Day 4 breakfast)<br><br>Handful of berries<br>Portion: 1 fruit | Grilled Skirt Steak with Radicchio and Ranch (page 125)<br>Portions: 1 protein, 1 fat<br>(serve leftovers for Day 4 dinner)<br><br>Cauliflower Fried Rice (leftovers from Day 1 lunch)<br>Portions: ¼ protein, ¼ fat, 1 vegetable | Lamb Koftas with Lemon-Tahini Sauce (page 140)<br>Portions: 1 protein, ½ fat<br>(serve leftovers for Day 5 dinner)<br><br>Garden salad with any Bone Broth Diet salad dressing<br>Portions: ½ fat, 1 vegetable |
| **Day 3** | Salmon Stacks (leftovers from Day 1 breakfast)<br>Portions: 1 protein, 1 fat<br><br>Handful of berries<br>Portion: 1 fruit | Stuffed Peppers (leftovers from Day 1 dinner)<br>Portions: 1 protein, ½ fat, 2 vegetable<br><br>Greek Cucumber, Tomato, and Red Onion Salad with Red Wine-Oregano Vinaigrette (page 166)<br>Portions: ½ fat, 1 vegetable<br>(serve leftovers for Day 4 dinner) | Cuban Pulled Pork (page 139)<br>Portions: 1 protein, ¼ fat<br>(serve leftovers for Day 5 lunch)<br><br>Braised Brussels Sprouts with Bacon (page 176)<br>Portions: ½ protein, 1 vegetable<br>(serve leftovers for Day 5 lunch) |
| **Day 4** | Soft-Cooked Eggs with Yucca "Soldiers" (leftovers from Day 2 breakfast)<br>Portions: ½ protein, ¼ fat, 1 starchy vegetable<br><br>Handful of berries<br>Portion: 1 fruit | Spicy Braised Chicken Thighs with Fried Capers (leftovers from Day 1 lunch)<br>Portions: 1 protein, 1 fat, 1 vegetable<br><br>Garden salad with any Bone Broth Diet salad dressing<br>Portions: ½ fat, 1 vegetable | Grilled Skirt Steak with Radicchio and Ranch (leftovers from Day 2 lunch)<br>Portions: 1 protein, 1 fat<br><br>Greek Cucumber, Tomato, and Red Onion Salad with Red Wine-Oregano Vinaigrette (leftovers from Day 3 lunch)<br>Portions: 1 fat, 1 vegetable |
| **Day 5** | Kimchi Omelet (page 96)<br>Portions: 1 protein, ¼ fat, ½ vegetable | Cuban Pulled Pork (leftovers from Day 3 dinner)<br>Portions: 1 protein, ¼ fat<br><br>Braised Brussels Sprouts with Bacon (leftovers from Day 3 dinner)<br>Portions: ½ protein, 1 vegetable | Lamb Koftas with Lemon-Tahini Sauce (leftovers from Day 2 dinner)<br>Portions: 1 protein, ½ fat<br><br>Kohlrabi, Jicama, and Carrot Slaw (page 167)<br>Portions: 1 fat, 1 starchy vegetable |

# Meal Plan
## Week 3

| | BREAKFAST | LUNCH | DINNER |
|---|---|---|---|
| **Day 1** | Shakshuka (page 97)<br>Portions: ½ protein, ¼ fat, 1 vegetable<br>(serve leftovers for Day 3 breakfast)<br><br>Handful of berries<br>Portion: 1 fruit | Sausage-Stuffed Eggplant (page 143)<br>Portions: ½ protein, ¼ fat, 1 vegetable<br>(serve leftovers for Day 4 lunch)<br><br>Garden salad with any Bone Broth Diet salad dressing<br>Portions: ½ fat, 1 vegetable | Not-Your-Mother's Meatloaf with Turnip Mash (page 128)<br>Portions: 1 protein, 1 fat, 1 vegetable<br>(serve leftovers for Day 3 lunch) |
| **Day 2** | Tropical Fruit Chia Pudding (page 99)<br>Portions: 1 fat, 1 fruit<br>(serve leftovers for Day 4 breakfast) | Seared Tuna Steaks with Jicama Salsa (page 151)<br>Portions: 1 protein, 1 fat, 1 fruit, 1 starchy vegetable<br>(serve leftovers for Day 4 dinner)<br><br>Garden salad with any Bone Broth Diet salad dressing<br>Portions: ½ fat, 1 vegetable | Pork Ragu with Zucchini Pappardelle (page 136)<br>Portions: 1 protein, ½ fat, 1 vegetable<br>(serve leftovers for Day 5 dinner)<br><br>Grilled Garden Salad with Green Goddess Dressing (page 164)<br>Portions: 1 fat, 2 vegetable<br>(serve leftovers for Day 4 lunch) |
| **Day 3** | Shakshuka<br>(leftovers from Day 1 breakfast)<br>Portions: ½ protein, ¼ fat, 1 vegetable<br><br>Handful of berries<br>Portion: 1 fruit | Not-Your-Mother's Meatloaf with Turnip Mash<br>(leftovers from Day 1 dinner)<br>Portions: 1 protein, 1 fat, 1 vegetable | Curried Cashew Chicken (page 115)<br>Portions: 1 protein, 1 fat<br>(serve leftovers for Day 5 lunch)<br><br>Garden salad with any Bone Broth Diet salad dressing<br>Portions: ½ fat, 1 vegetable |
| **Day 4** | Tropical Fruit Chia Pudding<br>(leftovers from Day 2 breakfast)<br>Portions: 1 fat, 1 fruit | Sausage-Stuffed Eggplant<br>(leftovers from Day 1 lunch)<br>Portions: ½ protein, ¼ fat, 1 vegetable<br><br>Grilled Garden Salad with Green Goddess Dressing<br>(leftovers from Day 2 dinner)<br>Portions: 1 fat, 2 vegetable | Seared Tuna Steaks with Jicama Salsa<br>(leftovers from Day 2 lunch)<br>Portions: 1 protein, 1 fat, 1 fruit, 1 starchy vegetable |
| **Day 5** | Mushroom and Scallion Egg Roll-Ups (page 103)<br>Portions: ½ protein, 1 fat, 1 vegetable<br><br>Handful of berries<br>Portion: 1 fruit | Curried Cashew Chicken<br>(leftovers from Day 3 dinner)<br>Portions: 1 protein, 1 fat<br><br>Cauliflower Rice Pilaf with Carrots and Pine Nuts (page 169)<br>Portions: 1 fat, 1 vegetable<br>(serve leftovers for Day 5 dinner) | Pork Ragu with Zucchini Pappardelle<br>(leftovers from Day 2 dinner)<br>Portions: 1 protein, ½ fat, 1 vegetable<br><br>Cauliflower Rice Pilaf with Carrots and Pine Nuts<br>(leftovers from Day 5 lunch)<br>Portions: 1 fat, 1 vegetable |

# Make Broth Fast with Your Pressure Cooker!

If you have a pressure cooker, it's extra easy to make a big batch of bone broth on your batch cooking day. Here's how to do it:

- Put all of your ingredients in your pressure cooker and add enough water to cover everything by 1 inch. Lock the lid of your pressure cooker in place.

- Set the pressure cooker over high heat until it reaches full pressure (about 10 to 15 minutes). Then reduce the heat to low and cook for 45 to 60 minutes if you're using chicken bones and about 2 hours if you're using beef bones. (Fish bones cook so quickly that pressure cooking isn't recommended.)

- When you're done, remove the pressure cooker from the heat and let it cool down naturally, until it's ready to open. When your broth is cool, just strain it and you're ready to go.

## PREPPING SHAKES—A BIG TIME-SAVER!

Want another great batch cooking idea? Prep some shakes ahead of time! Here's how to do it:

- Buy a high-quality beef protein powder. (Do not use whey protein powder, which is a dairy food.) Your best choice is a protein powder derived from pastured cows.

- Have enough glass jars or plastic bags ready for the number of shakes you want to make.

- Wash any fruits or vegetables you're using. Dry leafy vegetables. Cut fruit into small pieces and freeze on a baking sheet.

- Place enough fruit pieces and vegetables into each jar or bag to equal a serving.

- Label each jar or bag. You can also list the ingredients to add.

- Place your jars or bags in the freezer.

When it's time for your shake, just toss your fruits and veggies in the blender along with your other ingredients, and hit the "start" button. Voilà—in about a minute, you're done! And remember that shakes aren't just for breakfast or for your 7 p.m. snack on mini-fasting days. You can substitute a shake for any meal.

## STOCKING UP FOR YOUR 7 P.M. SNACKS

If you choose Plan 2 of the Bone Broth Diet, you'll substitute a snack for your last cup of bone broth at 7 p.m. Each snack should include:

- A serving of protein, about the size of your palm.
- A serving of nonstarchy vegetables (see Chapter 3), the size of a softball or more.
- A teaspoon of fat.

As you're shopping and batch cooking, make sure to plan for these snacks. For instance, set aside an extra chicken breast, some meatballs, or a burger, or purchase some smoked salmon or high-quality, additive-free deli meat.

Make sure you prep plenty of veggies for your snacks, along with a salad dressing that's ready to go. Salsa is handy, too—and it's easy to find additive-free salsa at the stores these days if you don't have time to mix up a batch.

Here are some fun ideas for your snacks:

3 to 4 ounces smoked salmon with sliced tomatoes and lettuce, drizzled with 1 teaspoon olive oil or 1 serving Balsamic Vinaigrette (page 80)

3 to 4 ounces cooked chicken breast, roast turkey breast, or whole roast chicken and steamed broccoli, drizzled with 1 teaspoon olive oil or ghee

1 turkey or chicken burger (3 to 4 ounces) wrapped in large lettuce leaves with 1 teaspoon Homemade Mayonnaise (page 76)

1 beef or bison burger (3 to 4 ounces) topped with your choice of salsa, plus a small salad of lettuce and tomatoes with 1 serving Ranch Dressing (page 84) or 1 teaspoon olive oil and vinegar or lemon juice

2 scrambled eggs with 1 teaspoon ghee and sautéed spinach

3 to 4 slices turkey breast (I recommend Applegate because it's free of sugar, nitrates, and gluten), 1 teaspoon Homemade Mayonnaise (page 76), and 3 to 4 asparagus spears to make roll-ups

2 to 3 cups mixed salad greens and other vegetables from the Bone Broth Diet vegetables list (page 35), topped with a small can of tuna or salmon with 1 teaspoon olive oil and lemon juice

2 to 3 cups mixed salad greens and other vegetables from the Bone Broth Diet vegetables list (page 35), topped with a sliced hard-cooked egg and Ranch Dressing (page 84)

## THINGS TO STOCK FOR YOUR THREE WEEKS

If you're following my meal plans and you want to make sure you have all the necessities, here's a handy checklist. Stock up now, and you'll be ready to go.

### Proteins

1 whole chicken, several legs and/or thighs, necks, and backs, and at least 6 chicken feet or 1 pig's foot for Chicken Bone Broth (in the freezer)

5 or more pounds of beef bones such as knuckles, joints, feet, and marrow bones, as well as 2 to 3 pounds meaty bones such as oxtail, short ribs, and shank for Beef Bone Broth (in the freezer)

Bacon—uncured, sugar-, dextrose-, nitrate-, and gluten-free

Canned anchovies

Chicken breasts (in the freezer)

Chicken thighs—bone-in, skin-on

Deli-sliced ham—sugar-, dextrose-, nitrate-, and gluten-free (Applegate brand)

Flank steak—grass-fed (in the freezer)

Fresh eggs

Ground lamb

Ground pork

Ground turkey (in the freezer)

Lean ground beef or ground bison

Pastured pork breakfast sausage (in the freezer)

Pork shoulder—boneless, skinless

Salmon steaks—wild, not farm-raised if possible (in the freezer)

Skirt steak—grass-fed (in the freezer)

Smoked salmon—sugar-, dextrose-, nitrate-, and gluten-free and wild, not farm-raised if possible

Tuna steaks—albacore or yellow fin

### Fats

Avocado oil (optional)

Coconut oil

Fresh avocados

Ghee

Olive oil

Sesame oil

### Vegetables

Any of your favorite precut and pre-washed vegetables

Bell peppers

Brussels sprouts

Carrots

Cauliflower

Chiles (optional)

Chives

Cilantro

Cremini mushrooms

Cucumbers

Dried porcini mushrooms

Eggplant

Fresh ginger

Garlic

Jalapeños

Jicama

Kale

Kohlrabi

Leeks

Plum tomatoes

Radicchio

Radishes

Red onions

Scallions

Several boxes/bags prewashed salad greens, such as baby kale, spring mix, romaine hearts, spinach, or arugula

Shallots

Shiitake mushrooms

Snow peas

Sweet potatoes

Turnips

Yellow onions

Yucca

Zucchini

## Fruits

Fresh berries—blueberries, strawberries, blackberries, and/or raspberries

Frozen berries—keep 2 bags in the freezer

Lemons—2 or 3

Limes—2 or 3

Mangoes

Oranges—3 or 4

Papayas

Pineapple

Tomatoes for salads—cherry, grape, heirloom, etc.

## Seasonings and Spices

Ancho chili powder

Any of your favorite fresh herbs, such as parsley, cilantro, basil, thyme, etc.

Balsamic vinegar

Bay leaves

Bell's seasoning

Cayenne pepper

Celtic or pink Himalayan salt

Cider vinegar

Coconut aminos

Crushed red-pepper flakes

Curry powder

Dried basil

Dried oregano

Dried thyme

Dry mustard

Garlic powder

Gochugaru (optional)

Ground allspice

Ground black pepper

Ground cinnamon

Ground coriander

Ground cumin

Ground nutmeg

Horseradish

Hungarian or sweet paprika

Italian seasoning

Red wine vinegar

Sherry vinegar

Sriracha sauce

Star anise

Unsweetened coconut flakes (optional)

Vanilla extract

## Canned, Jarred, Bagged, or Bottled Goods

Almond meal

Anchovies (also listed in proteins)

Capers

Cashews—raw, unsalted

Chia seeds

Chipotle chile peppers in adobo sauce

Coconut aminos (also listed under Seasonings and Spices)

Full-fat coconut milk—several cans

Kimchi

Red wine

Small cans (6 ounces) tomato paste—2

Tahini

Unsweetened coconut flakes (optional, also listed under Seasonings and Spices)

## NO-COOK MEAL OPTIONS

So far, I've talked about making your cooking easier on my diet. But what if you don't want to cook at *all*? If that's the case . . . no problem! Here are some easy tips for no-cook (and almost-no-cook) meals.

- Hit the salad bar at your local grocery store. Select cut-up veggies and lettuce and dress your salad with oil and vinegar. Then grab some hard-cooked eggs and some good sugar-free, nitrate-free, and gluten-free deli meat—again, I recommend Applegate. When you get home, combine your greens with your eggs and sliced deli meat, and you'll have a filling meal.

- Buy a rotisserie chicken and a bag of frozen precut veggies. Cook the veggies quickly when you get home, and you're all set.

- Reach for smoked salmon, canned salmon, canned tuna, or sardines. Presto: instant protein. Buy a container of fresh blueberries, some prewashed greens, tomatoes, a vinegar-and-oil dressing, and some tasty avocado to top your salad, and you're good to go.

- Make a shake! You can substitute a shake for any meal—not just breakfast. Make sure you load your shake with nutritious goodies like spinach, berries, or kale, and add full-fat coconut milk for a dose of healthy fat.

You can also eat out at restaurants, if you're willing to be assertive. Order plain grilled or roasted meat, chicken, or fish. Ask your waiter to leave off the bread, rice, potatoes, or pasta and instead give you a double serving of vegetables. Add a tossed salad, and you have a plate full of lovely "yes" foods.

To make eating out easier, select restaurants that cater to health-conscious people. Call them ahead of time and make sure they'll be willing to meet your needs.

## SHOPPING TIPS

One reason I recommend stocking your kitchen thoroughly before you start the diet is because grocery stores are filled with temptation—from cakes in the bakery to candy bars at checkout. The fewer trips you make, the fewer chances the Sugar Demon will have to woo you!

When you do go shopping, here are some rules that will help you stay the course:

- Stick as much as possible to the outside aisles, where you'll find your protein, fresh fruits and veggies, and butter. Think of the rest of the store as "enemy territory" and enter it only to grab a jar of olive oil, some coconut milk, spices, or other necessities. Don't go down the chips, cookie, and soda aisles at all, if you can avoid them.

- Eat a good meal before you head to the store. An empty stomach is the Sugar Demon's playground.

- Make a detailed list before you go, and stick to it.

- Read labels carefully. Even the most innocent-looking foods can have added sugar, flour, soy, or artificial chemicals.

- Shop at health food stores when you can. These stores are still filled with products containing soy, grains, and dairy, but they offer a better ratio of good food to bad.

And here's a final tip: If you're budgeting carefully, check the sales at your local stores before you shop. Frequently, you'll find organic chicken and beautiful organic veggies on sale (and turkey is dirt-cheap after Thanksgiving, while you can get bargains on lamb after Easter). This is a great opportunity to stock up for your batch cooking days!

# PART 2

# RECIPES FOR YOUR BONE BROTH DIET AND 80/20 PLAN

In this section, I'll introduce you to my favorite fat-blasting, skin-smoothing recipes—marvelous meals that turn dieting into a gourmet experience. Get ready to eat like royalty as you watch your wrinkles and extra pounds disappear!

One reminder: The "Make It a 20" recipes are for your 80/20 Plan, after you've completed your diet and lost all the weight you want to lose. When you reach this point, congratulations— now you can start sprinkling on a little "fairy dust."

## CHAPTER 5

# Building the Basics:

## *Your Bone Broth Diet Pantry*

THERE'S NOTHING HANDIER THAN a well-stocked pantry. And that's what this chapter is all about: filling up your Bone Broth Diet pantry! Only in this case, your "pantry" items are going straight into your fridge and freezer.

Of course, the first and most important food you'll want to have in plentiful supply in your chilly pantry is *bone broth*. After all, it's the core of your diet—the "secret sauce" that's going to melt off your pounds and erase your wrinkles. So in this chapter, you'll find four basic bone broth recipes plus five fun gourmet variations.

In addition, I've got you covered with the basic staples: healthy, diet-friendly versions of mayonnaise, ketchup, cocktail sauce, balsamic vinaigrette, and marinade. I even have two versions of pesto: a classic basil recipe and a different twist using broccoli.

I'll talk more about condiments shortly, and why you'll (usually) want to make them instead of buying them. But first, let's cover some bone broth basics.

## BUYING BONES FOR YOUR BROTH

To make the best bone broth, you need to start with the best bones—and here's how to do it.

First, get to know your butcher. This is the best way to get a good supply of knuckle, joint, foot, neck, and marrow bones—the bones that are richest in cartilage. If your butcher doesn't routinely carry these bones, you can special-order them.

If you can afford it, use bones from organic, pasture-raised animals. These bones have more nutrients and come from the healthiest animals. However, conventional beef bones are fine if you're watching your budget.

I throw in some meaty bones when I make broth, because they add extra flavor. Oxtail, shank, and short ribs are great choices. You can also add a cartilage-rich pig's foot to your beef broth to add more gelatin without affecting the taste.

By the way, I know the idea of throwing a cow's foot or a pig's foot in your stockpot may sound icky, but trust me, it will make your broth beautiful. However, you don't need to use feet if the idea grosses you out. You can make a fabulous broth using other cartilage-rich bones.

You can also collect bones from your meals and use them in your broth. It takes a while to gather enough bones for a batch of broth, but you can always add your leftover bones to the pot to augment the bones you buy.

For chicken or turkey bone broth, you can use any parts from the full carcass to necks, backs, and feet. Again, your butcher should be able to provide you with any cuts you want. Chicken feet are the best source of gelatin, but you might need to special-order them, and they're not a necessity. Just as with beef broth, you can add a pig's foot for more gelatin. I always add some whole chicken pieces for more flavor.

For fish, use the carcasses of low-fat white fish such as halibut, turbot, tilapia, cod, or rockfish. If you don't want to purchase the whole fish, see if your butcher or a local fish restaurant can save carcasses for you. Avoid oily fish like salmon and tuna, which can develop off flavors if you cook them for a long time.

Fish heads add great flavor and lots of gelatin to fish broth, and you can also toss in shrimp shells. Be very careful to keep a close eye on fish broth because it cooks quickly.

I want to stress one more time that it's *not* necessary to use any bones that make you squeamish—for instance, pigs' feet, cows' feet, chicken feet, or fish heads. You'll get plenty of fat-melting and wrinkle-erasing power from other cartilage-rich bones. But if you are adventurous and want to make a really gourmet broth, consider giving these "weird" options a try!

Of course, if you're in a hurry, you can obtain ready-to-eat bone broth—or even handy, portable collagen broth packets you can mix with water—from my Web site (drkellyannstore.com) or other sources. Just make sure you get high-quality broth from a source you trust.

## COOKING YOUR BROTH

Making bone broth is almost as simple as boiling water! It takes 5 to 10 minutes to throw a batch together, and after that, it will simmer away on its own. However, here are a few pointers for getting the best results.

First, your cooked broth should become bouncy when you chill it. If it doesn't, here are some troubleshooting tips:

- **Be sure to choose the right bones.** The bones need to be cartilage-rich, because it's the collagen in the cartilage that turns into gelatin when you cook your broth.

- **Don't "overwater" your broth.** If you dilute your broth too much, you may not get the jiggle you're seeking. When you make broth, barely cover the ingredients with water.

- **Keep the heat low.** It's best to keep your broth at a low simmer, barely bubbling. Also, put your pot on a small burner. If your stove temperature is too hot for the size of your pot, use a slow cooker, buy a bigger stockpot, get a stockpot with a heavier bottom, or keep the lid off or askew.

- **Watch the clock.** Follow the timing guidelines in each of the bone broth recipes so that you don't overcook or undercook your broth.

While jiggly broth is best, don't worry if your broth doesn't wiggle enough! It still contains loads of healing gelatin. If you want, you can add a packet of high-quality gelatin (I prefer Great Lakes brand) to your broth. Be sure to "bloom" the gelatin first according to the package directions, so it doesn't clump.

Another thing to know is that the vinegar in these recipes is there for a good reason: It helps to dissolve the bones so you get more nutrients out of them. And by the way, you won't taste it at all when your broth is done. You can use a little lemon juice in place of the vinegar if you'd prefer; it works in the same way.

## A NOTE ABOUT CONDIMENTS

You may wonder why I'm asking you to make your own condiments. If you check the labels on the jars in your pantry, you'll quickly discover the answer! Mayonnaise typically contains canola or soybean oil, sugar, and preservatives. Ketchup and cocktail sauce are loaded with sugar or high-fructose corn syrup. Pesto, in addition to frequently containing canola oil, also contains dairy. Even innocent-looking salad dressings and marinades can be loaded with sugar, artificial chemicals, or seed oils.

With a little searching, you can find salsas and salad dressings that contain only diet-friendly ingredients. Feel free to buy these—but they're also easy to make from scratch. In addition, there are a few healthy, diet-friendly versions of mayonnaise out there: Mark Sisson's Primal Kitchen Mayo and Chipotle Lime Mayo are great choices.

For the most part, however, it's wise to make your condiments from scratch. It's a handy skill to learn, and it allows you to have total control over your diet. Besides, I think you'll be surprised at how *good* fresh condiments taste. That's why you'll rarely find a bottle of ketchup or a bottled salad dressing in a professional chef's kitchen!

## *Making Clarified Butter (Ghee)*

When recipes call for butter, you'll use clarified butter. Here's a little info about what clarified butter is and how to make it.

When you remove the milk solids from butter, the remaining butterfat is clarified butter. Clarified butter stays golden yellow and doesn't separate. It also stands up better to high heat than unclarified butter does. (You can see why chefs love it!) On the Bone Broth Diet, it's important to clarify your butter so that it will be nondairy.

To make clarified butter, heat the butter gently; wait until the fat and dairy solids separate, and then spoon off the solids. Clarified butter will keep for 3 to 6 months in the refrigerator.

# CHICKEN BONE BROTH

This savory broth is loved the world over as a healing food, as well as the foundation for delicious soups, stews, and gravies. You'll find dozens of uses for it in my recipes, but it's also warming and satisfying straight out of the mug.

PREP TIME: 15 minutes
COOK TIME: 4 to 6 hours

YIELD: Varies depending on pot size (there are enough ingredients to make 1 gallon of broth)

3 or more pounds raw chicken bones/carcasses (from 3–4 chickens)

1 whole chicken

4–6 chicken legs, thighs, or wings

6–8 chicken feet or 1 pig's foot

¼–½ cup apple cider vinegar, depending on the size of the pot

Purified water to just cover the bones and meat in the pot

2–4 carrots, scrubbed and coarsely chopped

3–4 ribs celery, including leafy part, coarsely chopped

1 onion, cut into large chunks

1 tomato, cut into wedges (optional)

1 or 2 whole cloves

2 teaspoons black peppercorns

1 bunch fresh flat-leaf parsley

Place all the bones and meat in a large stockpot or slow cooker. Add the vinegar and enough purified water to cover everything by 1 inch. Cover the pot.

If cooking in a stockpot, bring the water to a simmer over medium heat. Use a shallow spoon to carefully skim the film off the top of the broth. If using a slow cooker, wait for about 2 hours until the water gets warm before skimming, but continue with the next step.

Add the carrots, celery, onion, tomato (if using), cloves, and peppercorns and reduce the heat to low. You want the broth to barely simmer. Skim occasionally during the first 2 hours. Cook for at least 4 hours or up to 6, adding water as needed to ensure the bones are always covered with water and adding the parsley in the last hour. (You will have to add water during the cooking process.)

When the broth is done, remove the pot from the heat or turn off the slow cooker. Using tongs and/or a large slotted spoon, remove all the bones and meat. Save the chicken for another recipe. Pour the broth through a fine-mesh sieve and discard the solids.

Let cool on the counter and refrigerate within 1 hour. You can skim off the fat easily after the broth is chilled, if desired. When chilled, the broth should be very gelatinous. The broth will keep for 5 days in the refrigerator or 3 or more months in the freezer.

# TURKEY BONE BROTH

Don't toss out that turkey carcass after dinner! Instead, turn it into this rich, satisfying broth—and be sure to try the broth in my Turkey "Pot Pie" (page 116).

PREP TIME: 15 minutes

COOK TIME: 6 to 8 hours

YIELD: Varies depending on pot size (there are enough ingredients to make 1 gallon of broth)

3 or more pounds raw turkey bones (backs and necks are usually available)

4–5 pounds turkey thighs or drumsticks

6–8 chicken feet or 1 pig's foot

¼–½ cup apple cider vinegar, depending on the size of the pot

Purified water to just cover the bones and meat in the pot

2–4 carrots, scrubbed and coarsely chopped

3–4 ribs celery, including leafy part, coarsely chopped

1 onion, cut into large chunks

1 tomato, cut into wedges (optional)

1 or 2 whole cloves

2 teaspoons black peppercorns

Place all the bones and meat in a large stockpot or slow cooker. Add the vinegar and enough purified water to cover everything by 1 inch. Cover the pot.

If cooking in a stockpot, bring the water to a simmer over medium heat. Use a shallow spoon to carefully skim the film off the top of the broth. If using a slow cooker, wait for about 2 hours until the water gets warm before skimming, but continue with the next step.

Add the carrots, celery, onion, tomato (if using), cloves, and peppercorns and reduce the heat to low. You want the broth to barely simmer. Skim occasionally during the first 2 hours. Cook for at least 6 hours or up to 8, adding water as needed to ensure the bones are always covered with water. (You will have to add water during the cooking process.)

When the broth is done, remove the pot from the heat or turn off the slow cooker. Using tongs and/or a large slotted spoon, remove all the bones and meat. Save the turkey for use in another recipe. Pour the broth through a fine-mesh sieve and discard the solids.

Let cool on the counter and refrigerate within 1 hour. You can skim off the fat easily after the broth is chilled, if desired. When chilled, the broth should be very gelatinous. The broth will keep for 5 days in the refrigerator or 3 or more months in the freezer.

# BEEF BONE BROTH

This broth is delicious all on its own—and it also stars in many of my favorite recipes, from Persian Lamb Shanks (page 135) to my Spicy Meatball Soup (page 183).

PREP TIME: 15 minutes
COOK TIME: 12 to 24 hours

YIELD: Varies depending on pot size (there are enough ingredients to make 1 gallon of broth)

4–5 pounds grass-fed beef bones, preferably marrow, joints, and knuckle bones

1 beef or pig's foot

3 pounds meaty bones, such as oxtail, shank, or short ribs

¼–½ cup apple cider vinegar, depending on the size of the pot

Purified water to just cover the bones in the pot

2–4 carrots, scrubbed and coarsely chopped

2 ribs celery, including leafy part, coarsely chopped

1 onion, cut into large chunks

2 bay leaves

1 or 2 whole cloves

1 tablespoon black peppercorns

Place all the bones in a large stockpot or slow cooker. Add the vinegar and enough purified water to cover everything by 1 inch. Cover the pot.

If cooking in a stockpot, bring the water to a simmer over medium heat. Use a shallow spoon to carefully skim the film off the top of the broth. If using a slow cooker, wait for about 2 hours until the water gets warm before skimming, but continue with the next step.

Add the carrots, celery, onion, bay leaves, cloves, and peppercorns and reduce the heat to low. Cover the pot. You want the broth to barely simmer. Skim occasionally during the first 2 hours. Cook for at least 12 hours or up to 24, adding water as needed to ensure the bones are always covered with water. (You will likely have to add water during the cooking process.)

When the broth is done, remove the pot from the heat or turn off the slow cooker. Using tongs and/or a large slotted spoon, remove all the bones and meat. Save the beef for another recipe. Pour the broth through a fine-mesh sieve and discard the solids.

Let cool on the counter and refrigerate within 1 hour. You can skim off the fat easily after the broth is chilled, if desired. When chilled, the broth should be very gelatinous. The broth will keep for 5 days in the refrigerator or 3 or more months in your freezer.

# Try Bone Marrow, Too!

Like bone broth, bone marrow is packed with healing nutrients—and it's delicious. Bone marrow is considered a delicacy in many cultures, and more and more fancy restaurants are adding it to their menus in the United States.

Here's an interesting historical fact: Specially shaped marrow bone spoons were very popular in Europe and England in the 19th century because they made it easy to scoop out and enjoy this delicacy.

## ROASTED MARROW BONES

PREP TIME: 1 MINUTE ● COOK TIME: 30 MINUTES

   1  or more pounds beef marrow bones
      Celtic or pink Himalayan salt
      Ground black pepper

Preheat the oven to 425°F.

Place the marrow bones in a shallow roasting pan and bake for about 30 minutes. Season with salt and pepper. Save the bones for your next batch of bone broth.

# FISH BONE BROTH

This delicate broth is a staple in Asian countries. It's featured in a number of my recipes, from Cioppino (page 180) to Mussels with Tomato and Fennel Broth (page 153).

PREP TIME: 15 minutes
COOK TIME: 1 hour 15 minutes

YIELD: Varies depending on pot size (there are enough ingredients to make 1 gallon of broth)

5–7 pounds fish carcasses or heads from large nonoily fish such as halibut, cod, sole, rockfish, turbot, or tilapia (see Tips)

2 tablespoons ghee

1–2 carrots, scrubbed and coarsely chopped

2 ribs celery, including leafy part, coarsely chopped

2 onions, coarsely chopped

Purified water to just cover the bones in the pot

1 bay leaf

1 or 2 whole cloves

2 teaspoons black peppercorns

1 tablespoon bouquet garni or small handful of fresh flat-leaf parsley and 4–5 stems fresh thyme

Wash the fish and cut off the gills if present.

In a large stockpot, melt the ghee over medium-low to low heat. Add the carrots, celery, and onions and cook, stirring occasionally, for about 20 minutes.

Add the fish and enough water to cover everything by 1 inch. Increase the heat to medium and bring the water to a bare simmer. Use a shallow spoon to carefully skim the film off the top of the broth. Add the bay leaf, cloves, peppercorns, and bouquet garni (or parsley and thyme) and reduce the heat to low. Cook at a bare simmer for about 50 minutes, uncovered or with the lid askew. Continue to skim the surface as needed.

When the broth is done, remove the pot from the heat. Using tongs and/or a large slotted spoon, remove all the bones. Pour the broth through a fine-mesh sieve and discard the solids.

Let cool on the counter before refrigerating. You can skim off the fat easily after the broth is chilled, if desired. When chilled, the broth should be very gelatinous. The broth will keep for 5 days in the refrigerator or 3 or more months in the freezer.

**TIPS:**

*It's important to use nonoily fish because the oils in fatty fish, such as salmon, can turn rancid in cooking.*

*The cartilage in fish bones breaks down to gelatin very quickly, so it's best to cook this broth on the stovetop.*

# THANKSGIVING TURKEY BONE BROTH

I call this broth "Thanksgiving in a mug." And you know what? I think I like it better than the turkey dinner!

PREP TIME: 5 minutes

COOK TIME: 5 to 10 minutes

YIELD: 4 cups (1 quart)

4 cups (1 quart) Turkey Bone Broth (page 66)

2 ribs celery, finely chopped

1 carrot, finely chopped

1 small clove garlic, smashed

¼–½ teaspoon ground sage or Bell's Seasoning (see Tip)

1 whole clove

Celtic or pink Himalayan salt

Freshly ground black pepper

In a saucepan, heat the broth over medium heat. Add the celery, carrot, garlic, sage or Bell's Seasoning, and clove. Reduce the heat to medium-low or low so the broth barely simmers and cook just until the carrots and celery are tender, 5 to 10 minutes.

Remove and discard the garlic and clove. Season with salt and pepper and serve.

TIP: *Bell's Seasoning is a salt-free blend of herbs and spices containing rosemary, oregano, sage, ginger, and marjoram.*

# Spice Up Your Broth

The herbs and spices in bone broth will tickle your tastebuds—and at the same time, they'll boost your metabolism, burn fat, and promote good digestive health. Here's a look at what some of these herbs and spices do for you.

*Ginger*: This warming spice has anti-inflammatory properties. It also soothes your intestinal tract. Ginger may have thermogenic properties that help boost your metabolism.

*Garlic*: A nutrient-dense food, garlic is rich in antioxidants. Allicin, a powerful antioxidant, is released when you smash, cut, or chew garlic. Garlic also reduces LDL cholesterol, which may lower your risk of heart disease. Garlic reduces oxidative damage from free radicals, slowing the aging process. It's been used medicinally for thousands of years. The ancient Greek physician Hippocrates, often called the father of Western medicine, prescribed garlic to treat a variety of medical conditions.

*Turmeric*: Curcumin is the active ingredient in turmeric. It slows the formation of fatty tissue and may contribute to reduced body fat and enhanced weight control. It is also an anti-inflammatory agent and reduces insulin resistance.

*Black pepper*: Piperine is the compound that gives pepper its pungent flavor. Piperine enhances the serum concentration, absorption, and bioavailability of curcumin, the active ingredient in turmeric.

*Cayenne pepper*: Capsaicin, the compound that gives chile peppers their heat, may help shrink fatty tissue and lower blood fat levels. Because capsaicin creates heat in the body, it may temporarily increase fat-burning.

*Cumin*: This herb aids digestion and is active in energy production in the body.

*Cardamom*: This is another warming, thermogenic spice that may help boost your metabolism and your body's ability to burn fat.

# ASIAN CHICKEN BONE BROTH

This light, lively broth features shiitake mushrooms, lemongrass, garlic, and cilantro. Between you and me, I think it's my favorite bone broth of all.

PREP TIME: 5 minutes

COOK TIME: 5 to 10 minutes

YIELD: 4 cups (1 quart)

- 4 cups (1 quart) Chicken Bone Broth (page 65)
- 1 length lemongrass (3 inches), cut into 1-inch pieces
- 1 small clove garlic, smashed

  Handful of shiitake mushrooms, sliced
- 2 scallions, white and green parts, cut into ½-inch pieces

  Celtic or pink Himalayan salt

  Freshly ground black pepper
- 2 tablespoons coarsely chopped cilantro leaves

In a saucepan, heat the broth over medium heat. Add the lemongrass, garlic, mushrooms, and scallions. Reduce the heat to medium-low or low so the broth barely simmers and cook for 5 to 10 minutes.

Remove and discard the lemongrass and garlic. Season with salt and pepper. Top with the cilantro.

# EASTERN EUROPEAN BEEF BONE BROTH

Shredded cabbage and dill give this broth an Old World twist. The cabbage helps to fill you up without adding carbs.

PREP TIME: 5 minutes
COOK TIME: 5 to 10 minutes
YIELD: 4 cups (1 quart)

**4 cups (1 quart) Beef Bone Broth (page 67)**

**1 small clove garlic, smashed**

**Large handful of shredded cabbage**

**1 rib celery, finely chopped**

**1 bay leaf**

**1 teaspoon dried dill**

**1 black peppercorn**

**Celtic or pink Himalayan salt**

In a saucepan, heat the broth over medium heat. Add the garlic, cabbage, celery, bay leaf, dill, and peppercorn. Reduce the heat to medium-low or low so the broth barely simmers and cook just until the vegetables are tender, 5 to 10 minutes.

Remove and discard the bay leaf, garlic, and peppercorn. Season with salt and serve.

# FRENCH ONION BEEF BONE BROTH

This broth's secret to success: The onions cook low and slow until they caramelize, giving them a rich, sweet flavor.

PREP TIME: 5 minutes
COOK TIME: 5 to 10 minutes

YIELD: 4 cups (1 quart)

4 cups (1 quart) Beef Bone Broth (page 67)

1 small clove garlic, smashed

About 1 cup Roasted Sweet Onions (recipe follows)

¼ teaspoon herbes de Provence

1 black peppercorn

Celtic or pink Himalayan salt

In a saucepan, heat the broth over medium heat. Add the garlic, onions, herbs, and peppercorn. Reduce the heat to medium-low or low so the broth barely simmers and cook for 5 to 10 minutes.

Remove and discard the garlic and peppercorn. Season with salt and serve.

## ROASTED SWEET ONIONS

PREP TIME: 10 MINUTES ● COOK TIME: 30 TO 35 MINUTES ● YIELD: 4 SERVINGS

3–4 large sweet onions, very thinly sliced into rounds

Celtic or pink Himalayan salt

Freshly ground black pepper

2 teaspoons coconut oil or ghee, melted

Preheat the oven to 350°F. Line 2 baking sheets with parchment paper.

Spread the onion rounds evenly on the prepared pans. Don't crowd the onions; you want them to roast and caramelize, not steam. Sprinkle with salt and pepper. Brush with the oil or ghee.

Bake for 20 to 25 minutes, turning the onions when the tops are golden brown, about half-way through the cooking time.

**TIP:** It's easy to pop these in the oven when you're roasting meat. If Vidalia onions are in season, be sure to roast some. They are unbelievably delicious!

# ITALIAN BEEF BONE BROTH

Basil, garlic, and tomato sauce make this broth *delizioso*. I like serving it as an appetizer when I have company for dinner.

PREP TIME: 5 minutes

COOK TIME: 5 to 10 minutes

YIELD: 4 cups (1 quart)

4 cups (1 quart) Beef Bone Broth (page 67)

1 small clove garlic, smashed

¼ cup no-sugar-added tomato sauce

¼ teaspoon Italian seasoning

Celtic or pink Himalayan salt

Freshly ground black pepper

6 fresh basil leaves, cut into a fine chiffonade

In a saucepan, heat the broth over medium heat. Add the garlic, tomato sauce, and Italian seasoning. Reduce the heat to medium-low or low so the broth barely simmers and cook for 5 to 10 minutes.

Remove and discard the garlic. Season with salt and pepper and serve topped with basil.

## *Need Bone Broth on the Run?*

Homemade stocks and broths tend to be much healthier than store-bought versions, which often contain MSG and other additives. However, on days when life is crazy, you may not have time to cook up a batch of bone broth. Luckily, it's now possible to buy dehydrated bone broth that has all of the nutritional value of liquid broth and is free of toxins and additives.

One big benefit of dehydrated bone broth is that it's portable. If you travel, you can carry on a lightweight packet of dehydrated broth when you fly and not have to worry about checking in a liquid. Also, if you or someone in your household has a sudden illness and you don't have any bone broth handy in the refrigerator, the dehydrated version can save the day.

If you buy dehydrated bone broth, make sure the broth is organic and the salt (if any) is mineralized salt or sea salt. If you can't find high-quality bone broth in a packet at your local stores, I offer it at drkellyannstore.com.

Also, remember that you want bone broth—not just regular broth or stock. Look for the word *bone* on the label.

# HOMEMADE MAYONNAISE

It takes only minutes to whip up a healthy, additive-free mayo in your food processor—and you won't believe how much better this condiment tastes when you make it fresh.

PREP TIME: 15 minutes

YIELD: about 1 cup or 16 portions

PORTION: 1 tablespoon = 1 fat

2 egg yolks

1 teaspoon Dijon mustard

1 tablespoon plus 1 teaspoon fresh lemon juice

Celtic or pink Himalayan salt

1 cup macadamia nut or avocado oil (olive oil is not recommended—see Tips)

Bring the ingredients to room temperature. Place the egg yolks in a food processor. Add the mustard, lemon juice, and salt to taste and pulse until the ingredients are completely combined. With the machine running, add the oil in a very slow, steady stream until the mixture is thick and emulsified.

Refrigerate in an airtight container. Because this is a fresh egg product without preservatives, use it within 5 days.

TIPS:

*Select very fresh, organic, free-range, properly refrigerated eggs with intact shells, and avoid contact between the yolks and the shell. If you feel more comfortable, use pasteurized eggs.*

*I don't recommend olive oil because it has a strong flavor that can overpower the delicacy of mayonnaise.*

**Variations:**

You can add a lot of pizzazz to mayo by introducing additional ingredients. There's no right or wrong way to add flavors to mayonnaise. Experiment, adjust the seasonings to suit yourself, and taste as you create.

**Roasted red pepper mayo:** Add about ½ teaspoon minced roasted garlic and about 2 tablespoons chopped roasted red peppers to ½ cup mayo. This works well, but remember, there are no rules. Trust your tastebuds! I like to leave bits of the roasted red peppers, but you can completely puree them. I also suggest adding about ⅛ teaspoon hot-pepper sauce (such as Tabasco) per ½ cup mayo to give it a little zing. A dash of cayenne pepper will work, too.

**Lime chipotle mayo:** Substitute lime juice for the lemon juice when you make the mayo. Add about ¼ teaspoon chipotle powder, ¼ teaspoon ground cumin, ¼ teaspoon minced garlic, and a dash of cayenne pepper per ½ cup mayo. Optionally, add 1 to 2 teaspoons minced fresh cilantro and/or ½ teaspoon grated lime peel.

**Herb mayo:** Add a combination of your favorite chopped fresh herbs, such as thyme, basil, dill, chives, marjoram, parsley, and cilantro. Optionally, add ¼ teaspoon minced garlic per ½ cup mayo.

**Aioli (garlic mayonnaise):** Add a few cloves of very finely chopped garlic to the food processor when you make the mayo.

**Hot and smoky mayo:** Use about ½ teaspoon chipotle chile in adobo sauce and ¼ teaspoon minced garlic per ½ cup mayo. Just as in the lime chipotle mayo, you can substitute lime juice for the lemon juice in the mayo recipe. You can also add ¼ teaspoon smoked paprika.

**Horseradish mayo:** Use ½ cup mayo and 1½ to 2 tablespoons prepared horseradish (from the refrigerated section of your grocery store) and a few twists of freshly ground black pepper. Optionally, you can add about ½ teaspoon finely chopped fresh rosemary. This is divine on beef.

# HOMEMADE KETCHUP

Five simple, natural ingredients are all you need to stir up this homemade ketchup in your own kitchen. Add a few more ingredients, and you'll have my Smoky BBQ Sauce (page 85).

PREP TIME: 5 minutes
COOK TIME: 5 to 10 minutes
YIELD: about 1 cup or 16 portions
PORTION: negligible fruit

½ cup tomato paste (sugar- and dextrose-free)

¼ cup apple cider vinegar

¼ cup unsweetened apple juice

Pinch of onion powder

⅛ teaspoon ground cloves

In a small saucepan, stir together the tomato paste, vinegar, apple juice, onion powder, and cloves. Heat over very low heat for 5 minutes, stirring constantly to prevent scorching. If you want the ketchup to thicken further, keep it at a very low simmer for a few more minutes.

Cool completely and store in an airtight container in the refrigerator for up to 2 weeks.

TIP: *Heating the ketchup encourages all the flavors to meld and will also slightly thicken it.*

# COCKTAIL SAUCE

Serve this spicy sauce with chilled shrimp or crab for a simple but classy appetizer. The bite of the horseradish pairs beautifully with the sweet flavor of the seafood.

PREP TIME: 5 minutes

COOK TIME: 5 to 10 minutes

YIELD: about 1 cup or 16 portions

PORTION: negligible fruit

½ cup tomato paste (sugar- and dextrose-free)

¼ cup apple cider vinegar

¼ cup unsweetened apple juice

Pinch of onion powder

⅛ teaspoon ground cloves

2–3 tablespoons prepared horseradish (see Tip)

Dash of hot-pepper sauce

In a small saucepan, stir together the tomato paste, vinegar, apple juice, onion powder, and cloves. Heat over very low heat for 5 minutes, stirring constantly to prevent scorching. If you want the sauce to thicken further, keep it at a very low simmer for a few more minutes.

Cool completely. Add the horseradish and hot-pepper sauce and stir. Adjust the horseradish and hot-pepper sauce to suit your tastes.

Cool completely and store in an airtight container in the refrigerator for up to 2 weeks.

TIP: *You can find prepared horseradish in the refrigerated case at the grocery store. The amount you need here will depend on how long you've had the horseradish opened, as it loses its potency over time. If your horseradish isn't fresh, you'll need to use the larger amount.*

# BALSAMIC VINAIGRETTE

This basic dressing brightens any salad. If you have an herb garden, try experimenting with different herb combos.

PREP TIME: 5 minutes

YIELD: about 1 cup or 16 portions

PORTION: 1 tablespoon = 1 fat

½ cup extra-virgin olive oil

½ cup balsamic vinegar

1 teaspoon dry mustard

½ teaspoon very finely chopped fresh thyme or ¾–1 teaspoon dried

1 clove garlic, smashed

⅛ teaspoon Celtic or pink Himalayan salt

In a bowl or jar with a tight-fitting lid, whisk or shake together the oil, vinegar, mustard, thyme, garlic, and salt. Refrigerate. Remove the garlic from the dressing before serving.

TIP: *This is best prepared ahead and refrigerated so the flavors can meld.*

# MY FAVORITE MARINADE

This versatile marinade is delicious with chicken, beef, pork, or seafood. It's an absolute must to have on hand during grilling season.

**PREP TIME:** 5 minutes

**YIELD:** enough for 2 pounds meat, poultry, or seafood

**PORTION:** negligible fat

- 1 tablespoon plus 1 teaspoon coconut oil, melted
- 3 tablespoons fresh lime juice
- ¼ cup coconut aminos
- 2 tablespoons finely chopped fresh ginger
- 2–3 cloves garlic, minced
- 1 teaspoon ground cumin
- ½ jalapeño pepper, seeded and finely chopped (wear gloves when handling)
- ¼ cup fresh cilantro, finely chopped
- ¼ teaspoon paprika
- ¼ teaspoon ground white pepper

In a bowl, whisk together the oil, lime juice, coconut aminos, ginger, garlic, cumin, jalapeño, cilantro, paprika, and white pepper. (Use a large nonmetallic bowl if you will be marinating in the bowl.)

# PESTO

Brushed on grilled shrimp, served with steak, added to scrambled eggs, or used as a meat marinade, this fresh green sauce adds a rich, nutty flavor.

PREP TIME: 5 minutes

YIELD: about 1 cup or 4 portions

PORTION: ¼ cup = 1 fat

2 cups tightly packed basil leaves

1 cup tightly packed baby spinach

2 cloves garlic, peeled

1 avocado, pitted and peeled

2 tablespoons pine nuts

1 tablespoon fresh lemon juice

½ teaspoon Celtic or pink Himalayan salt

In a food processor or blender, combine the basil, spinach, garlic, avocado, pine nuts, lemon juice, and salt. Process or blend until smooth, stopping a few times to scrape down the sides. Store in an airtight container in the refrigerator for up to 3 days.

# BROCCOLI STEM PESTO

Don't toss out those broccoli stems! Whirl them in the food processor with garlic, basil, walnuts, olive oil, and spices, and voilà: You have a fabulous pesto.

PREP TIME: 5 minutes

YIELD: about 1 cup or 4 portions

PORTION: ¼ cup = 1 fat

3 broccoli stems, coarsely chopped

1 clove garlic, peeled

1 cup basil leaves

2 tablespoons walnuts

¼ cup olive oil

1 tablespoon fresh lemon juice

½ teaspoon Celtic or pink Himalayan salt, plus more to taste

Freshly ground black pepper

In a food processor, combine the broccoli stems and garlic, and pulse a few times until chopped into small pieces. Add the basil and walnuts and pulse until finely chopped. Add the oil, lemon juice, and salt and pulse to combine. Season to taste with pepper and more salt.

# RANCH DRESSING

Who doesn't love this creamy, rich dressing? In fact, it's America's favorite salad topper—and you'll love it even more when you make it from fresh ingredients.

PREP TIME: 5 minutes
COOK TIME: 30 minutes
YIELD: about 1 cup or 16 portions
PORTION: 1 tablespoon = 1 fat

½ cup Homemade Mayonnaise (page 76)

2 tablespoons coconut cream (see Tip)

1 tablespoon chopped fresh dill

1 tablespoon chopped fresh flat-leaf parsley

1 small clove garlic, minced

1 teaspoon grated lemon peel

½ teaspoon onion powder

⅛ teaspoon Celtic or pink Himalayan salt

Pinch of freshly ground black pepper

In a bowl, mix together the mayonnaise, coconut cream, dill, parsley, garlic, lemon peel, onion powder, salt, and pepper until fully combined. Thin with 1 to 2 tablespoons water, if needed, to achieve your desired consistency; thinner for a dressing, thicker for a dip. Refrigerate for 30 minutes before serving. Store in an airtight container in the refrigerator for up to 1 week.

TIP: *Coconut cream is available wherever canned coconut milk is sold. If you can't find it, chill a can of regular full-fat coconut milk and scoop out the white part that solidifies at the top.*

# SMOKY BBQ SAUCE

This recipe, which starts with my Homemade Ketchup, adds heat from fresh jalapeños and smoked paprika and sweetness from apples. It serves up all of the flavor of a traditional BBQ sauce with none of the sugar.

PREP TIME: 5 minutes

COOK TIME: 15 minutes

YIELD: about 1¼ cups or 10 portions

PORTION: negligible fat

- 1 tablespoon olive oil
- ½ cup chopped onion
- 1 small jalapeño pepper, seeded (leave seeds in for more heat) and chopped (wear gloves when handling)
- 2 cloves garlic, minced
- 1 cup Homemade Ketchup (page 78)
- 2 tablespoons unsweetened applesauce
- 1 teaspoon smoked paprika
- ¼ teaspoon Celtic or pink Himalayan salt
- ⅛ teaspoon freshly ground black pepper
- ⅛ teaspoon chipotle powder

In a medium saucepan, heat the oil over medium heat until shimmering. Add the onion, jalapeño, and garlic and cook until softened, about 5 minutes.

Stir in the ketchup, ¼ cup water, applesauce, paprika, salt, pepper, and chipotle powder. Cook until thickened and slightly reduced, about 5 minutes. Remove from the heat, cool slightly, and then blend in a blender or food processor until smooth. Store in an airtight container in the refrigerator for up to 1 week.

**TIP:** *This sauce will taste best if made the day before so that the flavors can meld.*

# HARISSA

I never run out of ways to enjoy this fiery, garlicky Mediterranean paste. Add a little to burgers, use as a rub for meat or fish, serve with eggs, put a dollop in soups or stews, or mix with veggies before you roast them.

PREP TIME: 5 minutes
COOK TIME: 35 minutes
YIELD: about 1 cup or 16 portions
PORTION: negligible fat

4 ounces dried hot red chiles, such as ancho, New Mexico, guajillo, árbol, or a mix

1 red bell pepper

1 teaspoon caraway seeds

1 teaspoon coriander seeds

1 teaspoon cumin seeds

5 cloves garlic, peeled

2 sun-dried tomato halves

3 tablespoons fresh lemon juice

3 tablespoons extra-virgin olive oil, plus more for storing

1 teaspoon Celtic or pink Himalayan salt

Place the dried chiles in a heatproof bowl and cover with boiling water. Soak until softened, 20 to 30 minutes.

Over an open flame or under the broiler, char the bell pepper all over. Transfer to a small bowl and cover with plastic wrap until cool enough to handle, about 10 minutes. Using your fingers, peel away the charred skin and remove the stem and seeds.

Meanwhile, in a small dry saucepan, toast the caraway, coriander, and cumin seeds over medium heat, constantly shaking the pan, until lightly browned and fragrant, about 3 minutes. With a spice grinder or mortar and pestle, grind the seeds until fine.

Drain the chiles and transfer them to a food processor or blender with the roasted red bell pepper, garlic, sun-dried tomatoes, lemon juice, oil, spices, and salt. Blend until a paste forms. Season to taste with more salt or lemon juice. You can loosen the paste by adding more oil or a little water.

Transfer to a jar and top with a thin layer of oil to preserve the color and flavor. This will keep in the refrigerator for up to 1 month.

# CHIPOTLES IN ADOBO

Store-bought chipotles in adobo typically contain unhealthy ingredients including corn oil, cornstarch, and artificial colors. When you make this condiment from all-natural ingredients (including a dose of wrinkle-fighting bone broth), you'll get all of the rich, smoky goodness with zero guilt.

PREP TIME: 5 minutes

COOK TIME: 1 hour

YIELD: about 1 cup

PORTION: use as desired

7–10 dried chipotle peppers, stems removed and split lengthwise

1 cup strained tomatoes or crushed tomatoes

1 cup Beef Bone Broth (page 67)

¼ cup apple cider vinegar

½ small yellow onion, finely chopped

2 cloves garlic, minced

½ teaspoon Celtic or pink Himalayan salt

½ teaspoon ground cumin

¼ teaspoon ground cinnamon

⅛ teaspoon ground allspice

Pinch of ground cloves

In a medium saucepan, combine the chipotles, tomatoes, broth, vinegar, onion, garlic, salt, cumin, cinnamon, allspice, and cloves. Bring to a gentle simmer, cover, reduce the heat to low, and cook until the chipotles are completely softened, about 30 minutes.

Uncover and continue to cook until the sauce thickens, about 30 minutes more.

Let cool completely in the pan. Transfer to an airtight container and store in the refrigerator for up to 3 weeks, or freeze in ice cube tray portions for up to 3 months.

## MAKE IT A 20

*Add 2 tablespoons of honey to the mix to balance out the heat.*

## CHAPTER 6

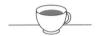

# Rise and Shine!

## *Beautiful Breakfasts to Start Your Day*

IS THERE MORE TO mornings than toaster waffles, Pop-Tarts, and cereal? Yes—and in this chapter, you'll discover just how satisfying it can be to eat *real* food for breakfast.

Even if your mornings are hectic, you can always make a healthy, delicious meal in seconds. When I'm in a rush, I toss a smoothie in the blender, warm up a bowl of soup, or grab one of my Coconut Almond Cranberry Fig Bars (you'll find the recipe in this chapter). You can't get much easier than that.

On a leisurely morning, however, I enjoy cooking up a scrumptious meal like Shakshuka, Pico de Gallo Eggs, or Sweet Potato Sausage Hash. And when my sweet tooth kicks in, I like to whip up a batch of my Flourless Banana Coconut Pancakes or my Tropical Fruit Chia Pudding. These are huge favorites around my house, and I think you'll love them, too.

### A WORD ABOUT EGGS

As you skim through my breakfast recipes, you'll notice that lots of them include eggs. That's because eggs are versatile, tasty, nutritious, and easy to cook.

However, if you've been listening to the authorities for years, you may be wondering: Is it safe to eat eggs frequently? Luckily, the answer is yes.

For decades, nutrition "experts" vilified eggs. They claimed that eggs raised your cholesterol, clogging your arteries and putting you at high risk for cardiovascular disease. But guess what: It isn't true.

We now know that while eggs contain a large amount of cholesterol, they don't raise your cholesterol significantly. In fact, when you eat eggs, your liver compensates by producing less cholesterol. So your overall cholesterol typically doesn't change very much; it's just that you're getting more from your diet, and less from your liver.

What's more, when eggs do change your cholesterol a little, studies hint that they do it in a good way. For instance, one recent study[1] found that for people with metabolic syndrome, eating eggs lead to a higher level of HDL (which is the "good" cholesterol) and beneficial changes in LDL (the "bad" cholesterol).

This is why experts are now singing a different tune about eggs. According to the newest draft of the Dietary Guidelines for America, "Cholesterol is not a nutrient of concern for overconsumption."[2] In plain English: Eggs are just fine for you.

In fact, eggs are more than fine—when it comes to nutritional value, they're amazing. For instance:

- They're loaded with protein, vitamins, minerals, and omega-3 fatty acids.
- They're one of the richest sources of choline, one of Mother Nature's most powerful fat flushers.
- They're excellent sources of lutein and zeaxanthin, which protect your eyes from cataracts and macular degeneration.

What's more, nearly all of these nutrients are in the yolk of the egg—the part those authorities told you to throw away! So take my advice: Keep your yolks, and toss out that bad advice instead.

## A BREAKFAST TIP: THINK OUTSIDE THE BOX!

While this chapter contains lots of egg recipes, you'll also find recipes that completely redefine the concept of breakfast. For instance, I've included everything from Salmon Stacks to Breakfast Turkey Burgers to Baked Sardines (sounds crazy, but it's delicious). You'll even find a Mediterranean Spaghetti Squash and Sausage Bake.

Remember: There's no law that says you have to eat "breakfast" food for breakfast! So get creative. Decide that *any* food can be a breakfast food, as long as it's a food that's good for you. True, your family may think you're nuts when they catch you eating sardines or turkey burgers at the breakfast table—but when they see your pounds melting away, I bet they'll throw out their toaster waffles and join you.

# HAM and EGGS TO GO

Want a delicious breakfast in a hurry? These grab-and-go muffins, filled to the brim with veggies, are just the ticket. Make them ahead of time, and refrigerate or freeze them.

PREP TIME: 15 minutes
COOK TIME: 40 minutes

YIELD: 12 muffins, 2 per serving

PORTIONS: 1 protein, ½ fat,
1 vegetable

- 4 tablespoons ghee or coconut oil
- ½ medium onion, chopped
- ½ medium red bell pepper, chopped
- 3 cloves garlic, minced
- 8 ounces cremini (baby bella) mushrooms, thinly sliced
- Celtic or pink Himalayan salt and freshly ground black pepper
- 8 ounces frozen spinach, thawed and squeezed dry
- 8 large eggs
- ¼ cup canned coconut milk, well stirred
- 12 slices deli-sliced uncured ham
- 1 cup cherry tomatoes, halved

Preheat the oven to 375°F. Grease a 12-cup muffin pan with 2 tablespoons of the ghee.

In a large skillet, heat the remaining 2 tablespoons ghee over medium heat. Add the onion, bell pepper, and garlic and cook until softened, about 5 minutes. Add the mushrooms and a pinch of salt and pepper. Cook, stirring, until the moisture from the mushrooms has evaporated, about 8 minutes. Stir in the spinach until warmed through and thoroughly combined. Set aside to cool.

In a bowl, whisk together the eggs, coconut milk, 1 teaspoon salt, and ½ teaspoon pepper. Stir in the cooled mushroom mixture.

Line each muffin cup with a slice of ham; there may be some overhang. Divide the egg mixture evenly among the ham cups. Top with the cherry tomato halves and bake until the egg mixture is set, about 25 minutes. Cool briefly, then carefully remove the ham cups to a rack to cool. Serve hot, warm, or at room temperature.

The muffins can be cooled completely and refrigerated for up to 3 days, or wrapped in plastic wrap and frozen for up to 2 months. To reheat, warm in a 350°F oven for 15 minutes.

# PICO DE GALLO EGGS

Give scrambled eggs a south-of-the-border twist with cilantro, jalapeño pepper, and a hint of lime. For extra heat, use a whole jalapeño instead of a half.

PREP TIME: 10 minutes
COOK TIME: 10 minutes
YIELD: 4 servings
PORTIONS: 1 protein, ½ fat

4 plum tomatoes, seeded and chopped

½ small red onion, chopped

½ jalapeño pepper, seeded and finely chopped (wear gloves when handling)

2 tablespoons chopped fresh cilantro

1 tablespoon fresh lime juice

Celtic or pink Himalayan salt

8 large eggs

2 tablespoons ghee

In a small bowl, combine the tomatoes, onion, jalapeño, cilantro, and lime juice. Season with salt to taste.

In another bowl, whisk together the eggs with ½ teaspoon salt.

In a large skillet, heat the ghee over medium-low heat. Add the eggs and shake the pan while stirring constantly, until large curds form, about 5 minutes.

Stir in the tomato mixture and cook until heated through and the eggs are to your liking, about 2 minutes more.

# SALMON STACKS

Looking for an elegant no-cook brunch idea? This smoked salmon dish is ready in minutes with almost no cleanup, and I love the combination of the cool salmon and cucumber, the punch of horseradish, and the bite of the radishes.

PREP TIME: 10 minutes

YIELD: 4 servings

PORTIONS: 1 protein, 1 fat

¼ cup extra-virgin olive oil

1 tablespoon prepared horseradish

8 small radishes, very thinly sliced

Celtic or pink Himalayan salt

½ English cucumber, very thinly sliced

12 ounces smoked salmon, thinly sliced

¼ cup thinly sliced fresh chives

Freshly ground black pepper

Lemon wedges, for serving

In a small bowl, whisk together the oil and horseradish. Set aside for the flavors to meld.

Shingle the radishes in a circle on 4 salad plates and sprinkle with a little salt. Layer on a few salmon slices, then top with the cucumber slices and a sprinkle of salt. Pile on the remaining salmon.

Drizzle with the horseradish oil. Sprinkle with the chives and pepper to taste. Serve with lemon wedges.

# SWEET POTATO SAUSAGE HASH

This new take on breakfast hash replaces potatoes with pan-roasted sweet potatoes, onions, peppers, and kale. It's a hearty, down-home breakfast—all in one skillet!

PREP TIME: 5 minutes
COOK TIME: 25 minutes

YIELD: 4 servings

PORTIONS: 1 protein, ¼ fat,
½ vegetable, 1 starchy vegetable

1 pound bulk pastured pork breakfast sausage

1 tablespoon olive oil

2 medium sweet potatoes, chopped

1 medium onion, chopped

1 red bell pepper, chopped

1 green bell pepper, chopped

½ bunch kale, ribs removed and leaves chopped

1 teaspoon fresh thyme leaves

½ teaspoon chopped fresh rosemary

½ teaspoon chopped fresh sage

In a medium skillet, cook the sausage over medium heat, breaking up the meat and stirring constantly until no longer pink, about 8 minutes. Remove the sausage from the pan, leaving any juices behind, and set aside.

In the same pan, heat the oil with any leftover juices from the meat. Add the sweet potatoes, onion, and bell peppers and cook until softened, about 10 minutes. Add the kale, thyme, rosemary, and sage and cook, stirring constantly, until the kale wilts, about 5 minutes more. Toss the sausage back into the pan and stir to combine. Serve immediately.

# SOFT-COOKED EGGS with YUCCA "SOLDIERS"

This fun finger food will make you feel like a kid again. Batons of yucca root substitute for toast dippers here, and hot sauce kicks up the soft-boiled egg.

PREP TIME: 5 minutes
COOK TIME: 25 minutes

YIELD: 4 servings

PORTIONS: ½ protein, ¼ fat, 1 starchy vegetable

1 medium yucca (about 1 pound), peeled and cut into ½-inch batons

1 tablespoon olive oil

1 teaspoon Celtic or pink Himalayan salt

¼ teaspoon freshly ground black pepper

4 large eggs

Gluten-free hot-pepper sauce (optional)

Preheat the oven to 450°F.

Bring a medium pot of water to a boil. Add the yucca and cook until tender, about 10 minutes. Drain well and spread in an even layer on a baking sheet, removing and discarding any woody cores. Drizzle with the oil and sprinkle with salt and pepper. Bake until golden and crisp, turning the yucca once, about 15 minutes.

Meanwhile, bring another medium pot of water to a boil, reduce the heat to a simmer, and slowly lower the eggs (in their shells) into the water. Cook for 5 to 7 minutes, depending on how runny you like your egg. Remove the eggs with a slotted spoon and run under cold water.

Place the eggs in egg cups and remove the tops using a knife to gently tap around the top of the egg. Serve the warm eggs with the yucca to dip in the yolk and hot-pepper sauce, if desired.

# KIMCHI OMELET

In this breakfast eye-opener, gochugaru-spiked eggs wrap around crunchy kimchi. A wake-up call for your tastebuds, and great for your gut as well!

PREP TIME: 10 minutes
COOK TIME: 10 minutes

YIELD: 4 servings

PORTIONS: 1 protein, ¼ fat, ½ vegetable

1 tablespoon coconut oil

1 small zucchini, halved lengthwise and thinly sliced crosswise

1 scallion, halved lengthwise and cut into 1-inch pieces

¾ cup chopped kimchi

8 large eggs

½–1 teaspoon gochugaru (see Tip) or crushed red-pepper flakes

Celtic or pink Himalayan salt

In a large skillet, heat the coconut oil over medium heat. Add the zucchini and scallion and cook, stirring, until the zucchini is slightly golden, about 3 minutes. Add the kimchi and warm through, about 1 minute.

Meanwhile, whisk together the eggs, chili flakes, and a pinch of salt.

Add the egg mixture to the skillet, cover, and cook until set, about 5 minutes. Slide onto a plate, slice, and serve.

TIP: *Gochugaru (Korean chili flakes) are used in Korean cooking and in kimchi. You can find them online or at an Asian market.*

# SHAKSHUKA (MIDDLE EASTERN POACHED EGGS)

This classic dish features eggs nestled in a bed of onions, peppers, and garlic sautéed with aromatic spices. It's a favorite around the world, and it's especially popular in Israel.

PREP TIME: 5 minutes
COOK TIME: 10 minutes

YIELD: 4 servings

PORTIONS: ½ protein, ¼ fat, 1 vegetable

- 1 tablespoon extra-virgin olive oil
- 1 large red or orange bell pepper, coarsely chopped
- 1 small yellow onion, coarsely chopped
- 1 clove garlic, minced
- 1 can (28 ounces) chopped tomatoes
- 3 tablespoons Harissa (page 86)
- ¼ teaspoon ground cumin
- ¼ teaspoon Celtic or pink Himalayan salt, plus more to taste
- 4 large eggs
- 2 tablespoons chopped fresh flat-leaf parsley

In a large skillet, heat the oil over medium heat. Add the bell pepper, onion, and garlic and cook, stirring, until tender, about 5 minutes.

Add the tomatoes, harissa, cumin, and salt and bring to a simmer. Crack the eggs into the sauce, leaving space around each; cover and cook until the whites are set, about 3 minutes. Season each egg with salt and garnish with parsley.

# BREAKFAST TURKEY BURGERS

Who says burgers are only for lunch or dinner? They're yummy, they cook in minutes, and you can mix up the ingredients the night before—making them a perfect breakfast food as well.

PREP TIME: 5 minutes

COOK TIME: 10 minutes

YIELD: 4 servings

PORTIONS: 1 protein, 1 fat

1 pound ground turkey

½ small onion, finely chopped

1 teaspoon dried sage

1 teaspoon garlic powder

¼ teaspoon Celtic or pink Himalayan salt

¼ teaspoon freshly ground black pepper

Coconut oil spray

1 avocado, pitted, peeled, and sliced

1 large tomato, sliced

½ cup alfalfa or radish sprouts

In a medium bowl, combine the turkey, onion, sage, garlic powder, salt, and pepper. Form into four 4-inch patties.

Spray a large skillet with the coconut oil spray and heat over medium heat. Add the patties and cook until a thermometer inserted in the center registers 165°F and the meat is no longer pink, about 5 minutes per side.

Serve the burgers topped with avocado slices, tomato slices, and a sprinkling of sprouts.

## MAKE IT A 20

*Serve with oven-baked home fries and Homemade Ketchup (page 78).*

# TROPICAL FRUIT CHIA PUDDING

Chia and coconut milk marry in a creamy pudding that pairs beautifully with fruit. In this recipe, I've gone tropical—but experiment with any fruits you like.

PREP TIME: 15 minutes

CHILL TIME: 1 hour

YIELD: 2 servings

PORTIONS: 1 fat, 1 fruit

⅔–1 cup canned coconut milk, well stirred

3 tablespoons chia seeds

1 teaspoon vanilla extract

½ mango, chopped

¼ cup chopped fresh pineapple

¼ cup chopped fresh papaya

Unsweetened coconut flakes, toasted (optional)

In a medium bowl or jar with a lid, combine the coconut milk, chia seeds, and vanilla and stir well. Cover and refrigerate for 1 hour or overnight.

Divide the pudding between 2 small bowls. Top with the mango, pineapple, papaya, and coconut flakes* (if using).

*1 tablespoon coconut flakes will increase fat to 1½ portions.

# COCONUT ALMOND CRANBERRY FIG BARS

You can make these easy, no-bake bars ahead of time. They're ideal for a quick breakfast, and they also make a perfect addition to a lunch box or hiker's backpack.

PREP TIME: 5 minutes

COOK TIME: 2 hours 5 minutes

YIELD: 16 bars, 1 per serving

PORTIONS: 1 fat, ¼ fruit

1 cup dried Black Mission figs

1 cup unsweetened shredded coconut

1 cup unsweetened dried cranberries

2 tablespoons coconut oil

1 tablespoon almond butter

½ teaspoon Celtic or pink Himalayan salt

½ teaspoon ground cinnamon

1 cup raw almonds

Line an 8 × 8-inch cake pan with parchment paper.

In a food processor, combine the figs, coconut, cranberries, coconut oil, almond butter, salt, and cinnamon and pulse until well mixed. Add the almonds and pulse until just combined.

Scrape the mixture into the prepared pan and spread evenly. Top with another sheet of parchment and press the mixture firmly into the pan with your hands or another cake pan, as evenly as possible.

Refrigerate for 2 hours. Cut into 16 bars. Store in an airtight container in the refrigerator for up to 2 weeks.

# MEDITERRANEAN SPAGHETTI SQUASH and SAUSAGE BAKE

In this simple but spectacular recipe, spaghetti squash serves as a base for an egg-and-sausage dish featuring the flavors of Italy. As an Italian girl myself, I can't get enough of this!

PREP TIME: 10 minutes

COOK TIME: 55 minutes

YIELD: 4 servings

PORTIONS: 1 protein, ½ fat, 2 vegetable

- 1 large spaghetti squash, halved lengthwise and seeded
- Coconut oil spray
- 2 tablespoons ghee
- Celtic or pink Himalayan salt and freshly ground black pepper
- 6 ounces Italian-style chicken or turkey sausage, casings removed
- 1 medium onion, chopped
- 2 cloves garlic, minced
- ½ teaspoon Italian seasoning
- 1 large tomato, chopped
- ¼ cup kalamata olives, pitted and halved
- 4 large eggs
- 1 cup baby arugula

Preheat the oven to 400°F.

Place the spaghetti squash halves, cut side up, on a large rimmed baking sheet. Spray each half with coconut oil spray and season with salt and pepper. Bake until tender, about 45 minutes.

Meanwhile, in an ovenproof skillet, melt the ghee over medium-low heat. Crumble in the sausage and cook, breaking it up with a wooden spoon, until no longer pink, about 5 minutes. Add the onion, garlic, and Italian seasoning and cook until the onion softens, about 5 minutes. Stir in the tomato, olives, and ½ cup water and simmer until saucy, about 5 minutes. Season to taste with salt and pepper.

Using a fork, scrape out the flesh from the spaghetti squash and add to the tomato mixture, tossing well to combine. Using a large spoon, make 4 deep wells in the mixture and crack an egg into each. Transfer the skillet to the oven and bake until the egg whites are set, about 7 minutes.

Serve topped with arugula.

# FLOURLESS BANANA COCONUT PANCAKES with BERRY SYRUP

You'll be ready to kiss heavy, carb-laden pancakes goodbye when you taste this light, fruit-filled alternative. It's pancake paradise—and every bite is good for you.

PREP TIME: 5 minutes
COOK TIME: 25 minutes

YIELD: 6 servings, 2 pancakes each

PORTIONS: ¼ protein, ¼ fat, 2 fruit

1 lemon

3 cups frozen mixed berries, such as blueberries, strawberries, and raspberries

3 medium firm-ripe bananas

3 large eggs

⅓ cup unsweetened shredded coconut

½ teaspoon baking powder

¼ teaspoon Celtic or pink Himalayan salt

3 tablespoons coconut oil

Grate the peel from the lemon and squeeze the juice. (You'll need 1 teaspoon peel and 2 tablespoons juice.)

In a medium saucepan, combine the berries and lemon juice and bring to a boil over medium-high heat. Reduce the heat to low and continue cooking, mashing the berries with a fork, until the berries are tender and have thickened slightly, about 10 minutes. Remove from the heat and set aside.

In a blender, combine the bananas, eggs, coconut, lemon peel, baking powder, and salt and puree until smooth.

In a large skillet, heat 1 tablespoon of the coconut oil over medium-high heat. Pour a few scant ¼ cups of batter into the pan and cook until the bottoms are golden and the tops are set, about 3 minutes. Turn and cook until cooked through, about 2 minutes more. Repeat with the remaining oil and batter.

Serve topped with the warm berry syrup.

# MUSHROOM and SCALLION EGG ROLL-UPS

This lovely dish stars eggs cooked crepe-style and rolled around sautéed mushrooms and scallions. I like to serve this for breakfast when company comes, because it always makes a big impression.

PREP TIME: 5 minutes

COOK TIME: 25 minutes

YIELD: 4 servings

PORTIONS: ½ protein, 1 fat, 1 vegetable

¼ cup ghee

8 ounces sliced shiitake caps

2 scallions, thinly sliced

1 clove garlic, minced

Celtic or pink Himalayan salt and freshly ground black pepper

4 large eggs

In a small (8-inch) skillet, heat 2 teaspoons of the ghee over medium heat. Add the mushrooms, scallions, garlic, and a pinch of salt and pepper. Cook, stirring, until the mushrooms are golden around the edges, about 8 minutes. Transfer to a bowl and keep warm.

Crack an egg into a bowl and whisk thoroughly with a pinch of salt and pepper. In the same pan, melt 2 teaspoons of the ghee over medium-low heat and pour in the beaten egg, swirling the pan to spread out to the edges. Cook until set, about 2 minutes. Top with one-quarter of the mushroom mixture and roll onto a plate. Repeat with the remaining ghee, eggs, and mushroom mixture.

# BAKED SARDINES with EGGS

Victorian breakfasts frequently featured a fish dish—and when you taste this, you'll know that they had the right idea. I'm delighted to play a part in bringing back this healthy and delicious tradition.

PREP TIME: 10 minutes

COOK TIME: 25 minutes

YIELD: 3 servings

PORTIONS: 1 protein, ½ fat

1 can (4.4 ounces) olive oil–packed sardines, broken into pieces (oil reserved)

1 large shallot, thinly sliced

¼ cup finely chopped fresh flat-leaf parsley

4 cloves garlic, minced

1 tablespoon fresh lemon juice

¼ teaspoon freshly ground black pepper, plus more to taste

6 large eggs

Celtic or pink Himalayan salt

Gluten-free hot-pepper sauce or salsa (optional)

Preheat the oven to 500°F. Set a large metal baking dish in the oven for 5 minutes.

Meanwhile, in a medium bowl, mix the sardines and their oil with the shallot, parsley, garlic, lemon juice, and pepper. Remove the dish from the oven and carefully add the sardine mixture. Return to the oven and bake until the shallot and garlic soften, about 6 minutes.

Take the dish out of the oven. Gently crack the eggs over the sardines. Season to taste with salt and pepper and return the dish to the oven. Bake until the egg whites are set, 5 to 7 minutes. Remove from the oven and set aside for 4 to 5 minutes so the eggs finish cooking. Serve with hot-pepper sauce or salsa, if desired.

## CHAPTER 7

# Main Course Magic:

## *Enticing Entrees for Lunch and Dinner*

YOU KNOW WHAT I remember most about my own days on low-calorie, low-fat diets? Eyeing my friends' luscious entrees longingly as I picked at a limp-lettuce-and-dry-chicken salad and tried to convince myself that I wasn't starving.

Well, guess what: Those days are over! Now, I feast on amazing foods like Chicken Cacciatore, Lamb Koftas, and Short Ribs with Salsa Verde. Every meal is a delight—and every entree is loaded with nutrients that keep my skin young and my figure slim.

In this chapter, I'll share dozens of my sensational entrees starring chicken, turkey, beef, lamb, pork, and fish. In addition, I'm including vegetarian entrees that even nonvegetarians will love. You'll find something for every taste, every budget, and every person in your life.

## SOME STRAIGHT TALK ABOUT PROTEINS

One question some of my patients ask when they see my entree recipes is, "Isn't this diet too high in protein?" If that's a concern for you, let me reassure you: The answer is a big *no*.

Here's the reality. The low-fat, low-calorie diets you're used to are often danger-ously *low* in protein. And low-carb diets that tell you to eat unlimited amounts of protein—for instance, a double burger with cheese and bacon for lunch—are dan-gerously *high* in protein.

In contrast, my diet is a *moderate-protein diet*. And I don't want you to short your-self on that protein, because it does great things for your body. Protein revs up your metabolism, speeding your weight loss. It also fills you up, so you don't crave sweets and carbs. And it's loaded with nutrients like fat-burning choline, conjugated lin-oleic acid (CLA), and skin-smoothing omega-3 fatty acids. (By the way, if you're worried about saturated fat, I'll tell you later on why you shouldn't be.)

Remember my rule of thumb: A serving of protein should be about the size and thickness of your palm. This ensures that you get all the nutrients you need from protein, without overdoing it.

So enjoy those beautiful proteins every day—your body will thank you for it!

# Chicken/Poultry

I love poultry because it's so versatile and easy to cook. Roast a couple of chickens or a turkey breast on your batch cooking days, and you can turn your bounty into everything from my Mediterranean Plate to my no-grain Turkey "Pot Pie."

And here's a bonus: If you want to go organic but have a limited budget, you can often find cheap chicken cuts. Organic chicken legs, in particular, are inexpensive. (However, don't fret if you can't afford organic chicken. It's not a deal-breaker at all! Simply remove the skin if you're using nonorganic chicken.)

Oh, and don't forget: You can save even more pennies by collecting the bones after you serve the delicious entrees in this section, and saving them for your next batch of bone broth. How's that for recycling?

# ASIAN CHICKEN HASH

Hash doesn't need to mean meat and potatoes! Try this very different version, infused with Asian flavors and loaded with chicken and fresh veggies.

PREP TIME: 10 minutes
COOK TIME: 10 minutes
YIELD: 4 servings
PORTIONS: 1 protein, ¼ fat, 1 vegetable

2 teaspoons rice vinegar

1 teaspoon toasted sesame oil

½ teaspoon grated fresh ginger

½ teaspoon Celtic or pink Himalayan salt

¼ teaspoon freshly ground black pepper

1 teaspoon coconut oil

½ napa cabbage, shredded

½ cup snow peas, trimmed

3 scallions, minced

4 cups shredded cooked chicken

Toasted sesame seeds, for garnish

In a small bowl, stir together the vinegar, sesame oil, ginger, salt, and pepper.

In a wok or large pan, heat the coconut oil over medium-high heat. Add the cabbage, snow peas, and scallions and cook until wilted, about 5 minutes.

Stir in the chicken and cook until heated through, 2 minutes more. Add the sesame oil mixture to the pan and toss to coat all the ingredients. Serve immediately, garnished with toasted sesame seeds.

# PECAN-CRUSTED CHICKEN with HOMESTYLE APPLESAUCE

Elevate your chicken breast with a crunchy nut crust. Chunky, cinnamon-spiced applesauce makes a sweet side.

PREP TIME: 10 minutes

COOK TIME: 25 minutes

YIELD: 4 servings

PORTIONS: 1 protein, ½ fat, 1 fruit

**For the applesauce:**

- 2 apples, such as McIntosh or Golden Delicious, peeled (see Tip), cored, and cut into ½- to 1-inch chunks
- Pinch of ground cinnamon

**For the chicken:**

- 1 pound boneless, skinless chicken breasts
- 1 teaspoon Celtic or pink Himalayan salt
- 1 teaspoon freshly ground black pepper
- 1 large egg
- ½ cup ground or very finely chopped pecans
- 2 tablespoons olive or coconut oil

*For the applesauce:* In a medium saucepan, combine the apples, 2 tablespoons water, and the cinnamon. Cover and cook over medium-low heat until the apples are very tender, about 25 minutes. Stir to smash the apples into a chunky sauce. Cover and set aside to keep warm. Stir before using.

*For the chicken:* Cut each breast crosswise into thirds. Place the pieces between 2 sheets of plastic wrap or in a zip-top plastic bag and pound with a meat mallet or heavy skillet until an even ½ inch thick. Season the pieces with ½ teaspoon of the salt and ½ teaspoon of the pepper. Set aside.

In a shallow bowl or pie plate, lightly beat the egg with ¼ teaspoon of the salt and ¼ teaspoon of the pepper. In a separate bowl, combine the pecans and the remaining ¼ teaspoon each salt and pepper.

Dip each cutlet into the egg mixture, evenly coating both sides and allowing excess egg to drip off. Dredge in the pecan mixture, pressing lightly to coat both sides.

In a skillet, heat 1 tablespoon of the oil over medium heat. Add half the chicken and cook until deep golden on both sides and no longer pink, about 5 minutes per side. Wipe out the pan and repeat with the remaining oil and chicken.

Serve with the warm applesauce.

**TIP:** *For added fiber, leave the peel on the apples when making the applesauce.*

# CHICKEN CACCIATORE

In this easy one-pot meal, skinless chicken thighs simmer in a garlicky tomato, caper, and mushroom sauce. Because it takes just minutes to prep, this is one of my favorite go-to meals for busy weeknights.

PREP TIME: 10 minutes

COOK TIME: 40 minutes

YIELD: 4 servings

PORTIONS: 1 protein, ½ fat, 1 vegetable

2 tablespoons olive oil

4 boneless, skinless chicken thighs

2 cups sliced mushrooms

1 medium onion, finely chopped

2 cloves garlic, minced

1 can (15 ounces) diced tomatoes

1 cup Chicken Bone Broth (page 65)

2 tablespoons capers, rinsed and drained

1 teaspoon dried oregano

1 teaspoon dried basil

½ teaspoon Celtic or pink Himalayan salt

¼ teaspoon freshly ground black pepper

Fresh basil, for garnish

In a large skillet, heat the oil over medium-high heat until shimmering. Add the chicken thighs and cook until golden, about 6 minutes per side. Remove from the skillet and set aside.

To the same skillet, add the mushrooms, onion, and garlic and cook until softened, about 5 minutes. Add the tomatoes, broth, capers, oregano, basil, salt, and pepper and bring to a simmer.

Return the chicken to the skillet, reduce the heat, cover, and cook until a thermometer inserted in a chicken thigh registers 165°F, about 20 minutes. Serve the chicken with the tomato broth and veggies, garnished with fresh basil.

# CHICKEN TIKKA

Marinate bite-size chunks of chicken in a creamy sauce packed with aromatic Indian spices, then thread them on skewers for a quick grilling. You can also cook the skewers under the oven broiler or in a grill pan.

PREP TIME: 10 minutes
COOK TIME: 10 minutes plus 1 hour marinating time
YIELD: 4 servings
PORTIONS: 1 protein, ½ fat

- 3 tablespoons cilantro leaves, plus more for garnish
- 2 tablespoons fresh lemon juice
- 2 cloves garlic, peeled
- 1 small fresh Thai chile, seeded (wear gloves when handling)
- 1 piece fresh ginger (1 inch), peeled
- 1 teaspoon ground turmeric
- ½ teaspoon ground cumin
- ½ teaspoon garam masala
- Celtic or pink Himalayan salt
- ½ cup coconut milk
- 1½ pounds boneless, skinless chicken breasts, cut into 1-inch pieces
- 8 bamboo skewers (12 inches), soaked in water for 30 minutes and dried
- 1 pint heirloom cherry tomatoes
- Freshly ground black pepper
- 2 tablespoons ghee
- Lemon wedges, for serving

In a mini food processor, combine the cilantro, lemon juice, garlic, chile, ginger, turmeric, cumin, garam masala, and 1 teaspoon salt and pulse to a smooth paste.

Transfer the paste to a large bowl, stir in the coconut milk, and toss in the chicken, mixing to coat completely. Cover and marinate in the refrigerator for 1 hour.

Preheat a gas or charcoal grill to medium-high heat. Brush the grates with avocado oil.

Thread the marinated chicken onto the skewers, adding a tomato between every 2 pieces of chicken and leaving space between the pieces. Season with salt and pepper.

Warm the ghee until liquid. Grill the skewers, turning and basting with the ghee every 2 to 3 minutes, until the chicken is no longer pink and the juices run clear, about 10 minutes total.

Transfer the skewers to a serving platter. Garnish with cilantro and lemon wedges.

# TURKEY KALE MEATBALLS with ZUCCHINI NOODLES and SALSA CRUDA

These meatballs bake while you prep your "zoodles" and make a fresh, no-cook salsa. I like to double the meatballs when I make this recipe so I have a head start on a second dinner.

PREP TIME: 20 minutes

COOK TIME: 20 minutes

YIELD: 4 servings

PORTIONS: 1 protein, ½ fat, 2 vegetable

**For the meatballs:**

1 pound ground turkey

10 ounces frozen kale, thawed

½ cup minced yellow onion

½ cup grated carrot

2 large egg whites

1 clove garlic, minced

Celtic or pink Himalayan salt and freshly ground black pepper

**For the salsa cruda and noodles:**

3 tomatoes, coarsely chopped

½ medium yellow onion, chopped

1 clove garlic, minced

2 tablespoons extra-virgin olive oil

1 tablespoon balsamic vinegar

3 medium zucchini, spiralized or peeled

2 tablespoons thinly sliced basil leaves

*For the meatballs:* Position a rack in the center of the oven and preheat to 425°F. Line a large rimmed baking sheet with foil and coat with coconut oil spray.

In a large bowl, combine the turkey, kale, onion, carrot, egg whites, garlic, and a pinch of salt and pepper. With wet hands, form 12 meatballs the size of golf balls. Place on the prepared baking sheet and coat with a bit more coconut oil spray. Bake until no longer pink and lightly golden, turning the meatballs halfway through, about 18 minutes.

*Meanwhile, for the salsa and noodles:* In a medium bowl, toss together the tomatoes, onion, garlic, oil, and vinegar. Season to taste with salt and pepper.

Divide the zucchini noodles among 4 plates. Top with the salsa cruda, 3 meatballs each, and a sprinkling of basil.

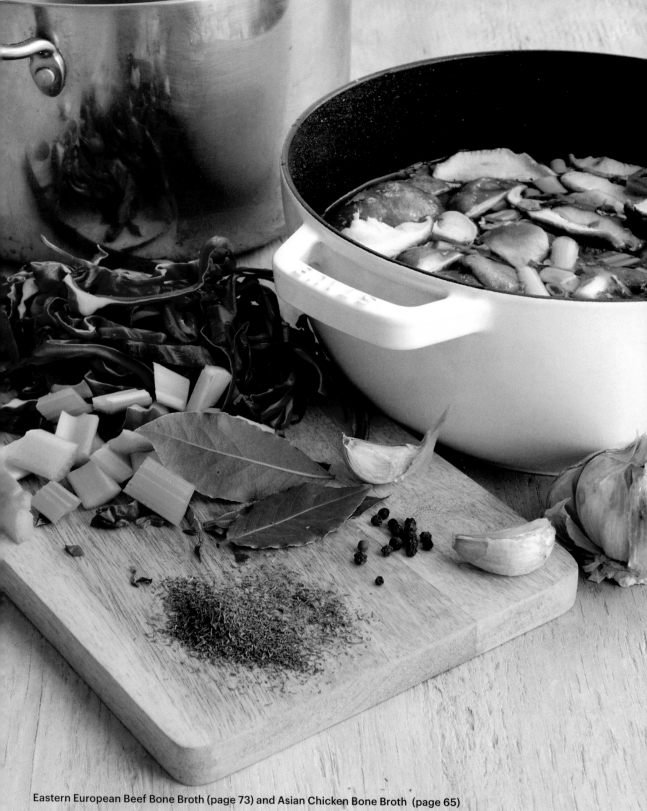

Eastern European Beef Bone Broth (page 73) and Asian Chicken Bone Broth (page 65)

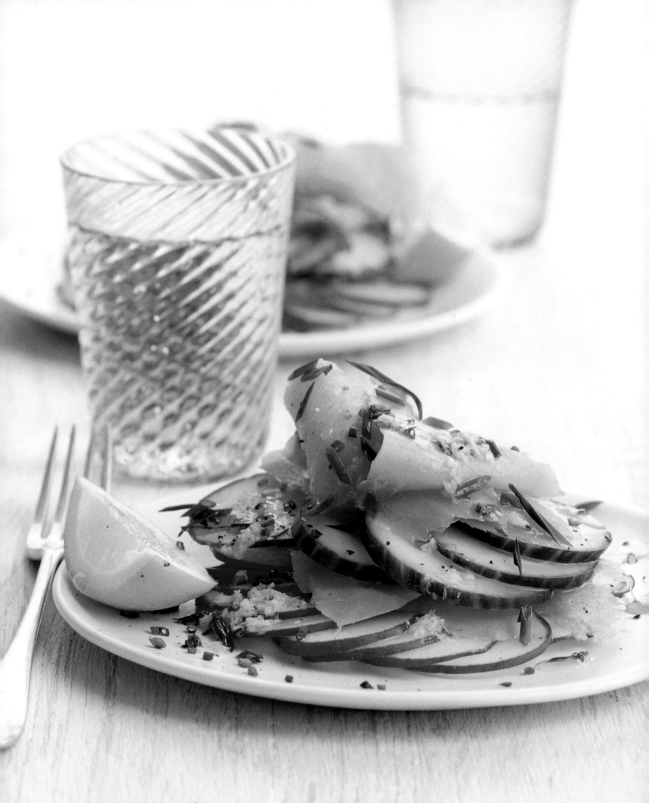

Salmon Stacks (page 93)

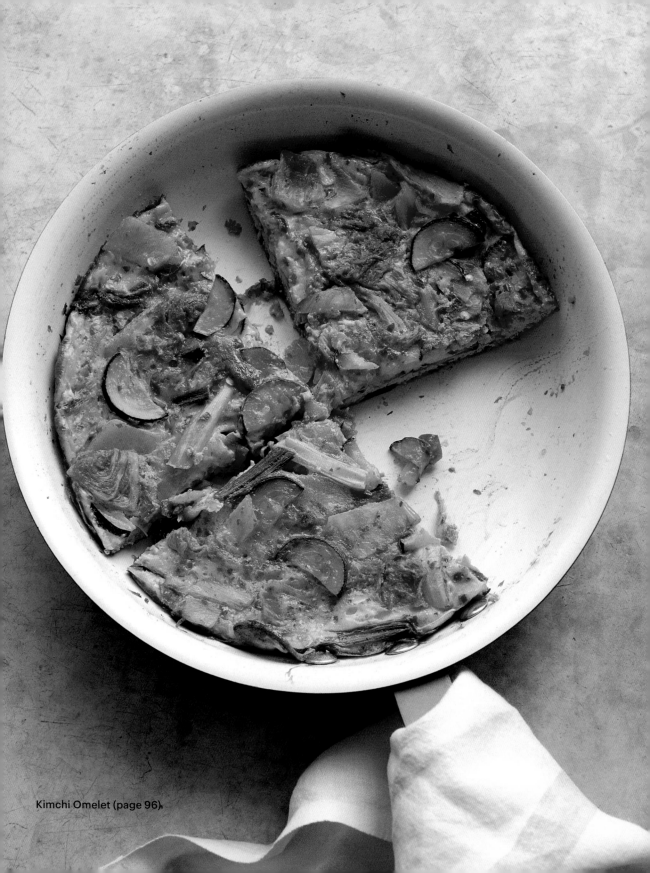

Kimchi Omelet (page 96)

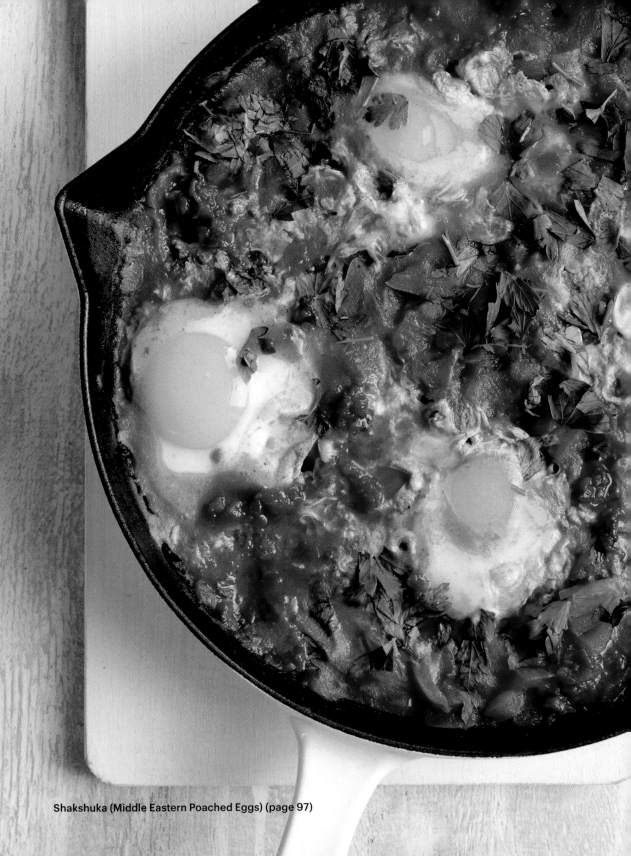

Shakshuka (Middle Eastern Poached Eggs) (page 97)

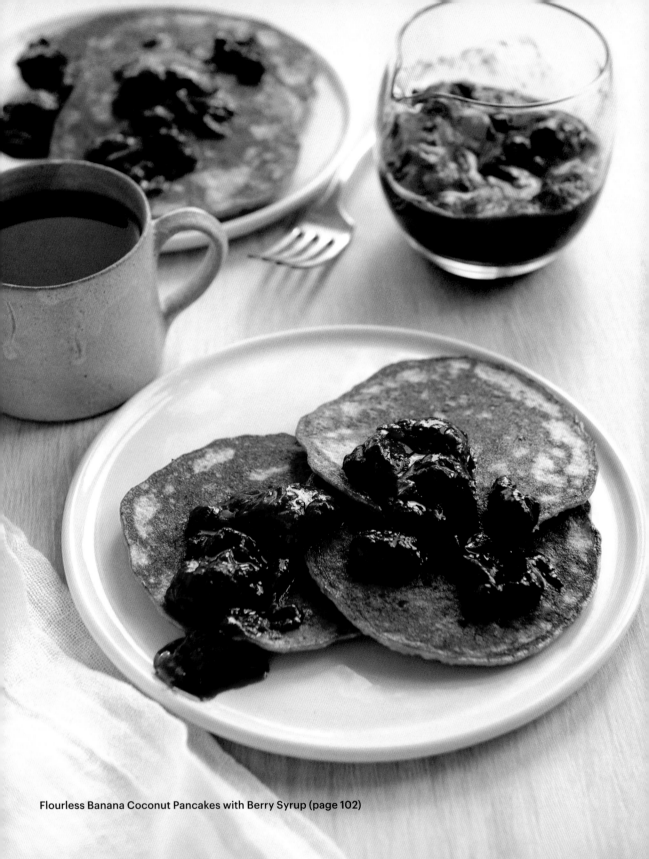

Flourless Banana Coconut Pancakes with Berry Syrup (page 102)

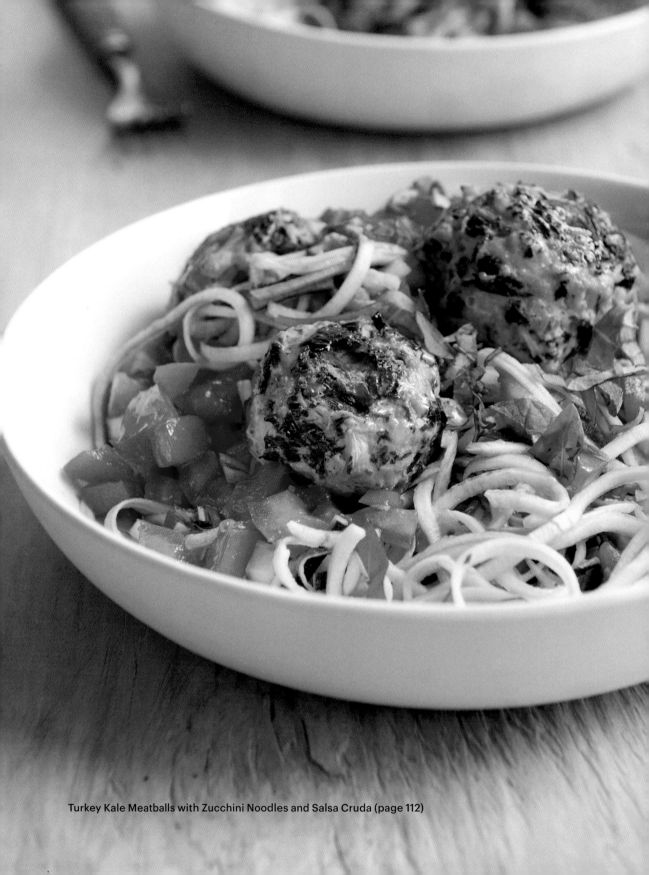

Turkey Kale Meatballs with Zucchini Noodles and Salsa Cruda (page 112)

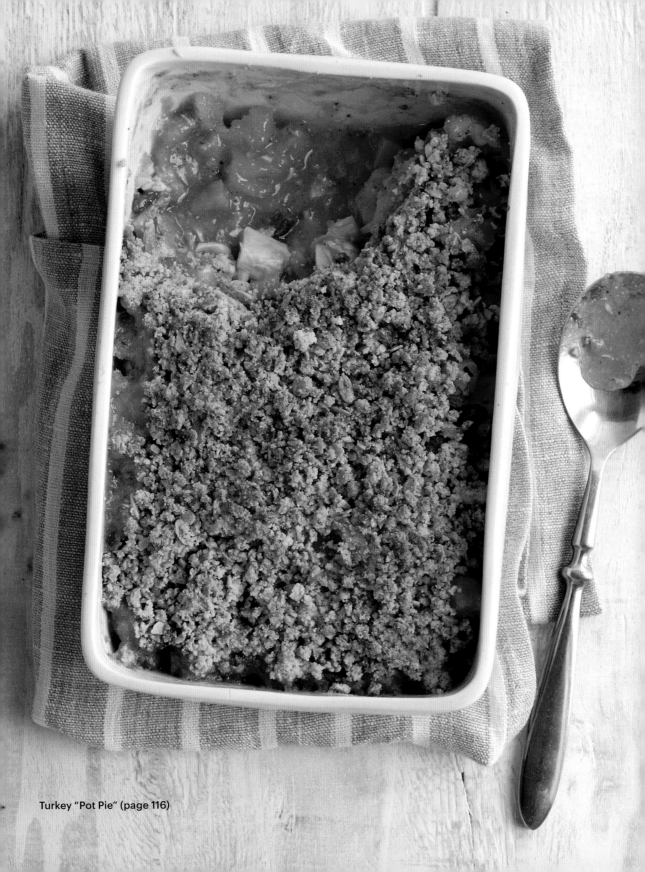

Turkey "Pot Pie" (page 116)

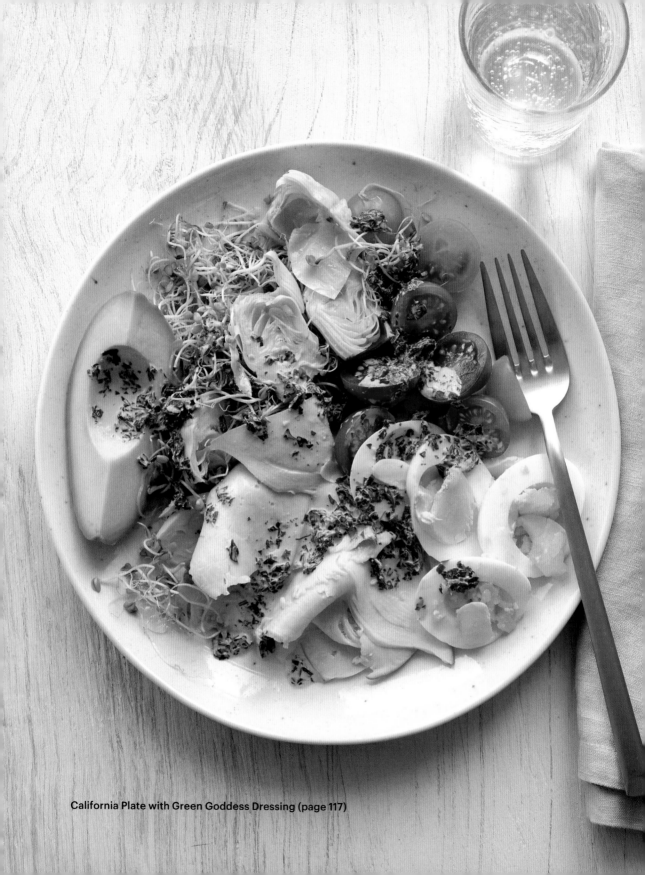

California Plate with Green Goddess Dressing (page 117)

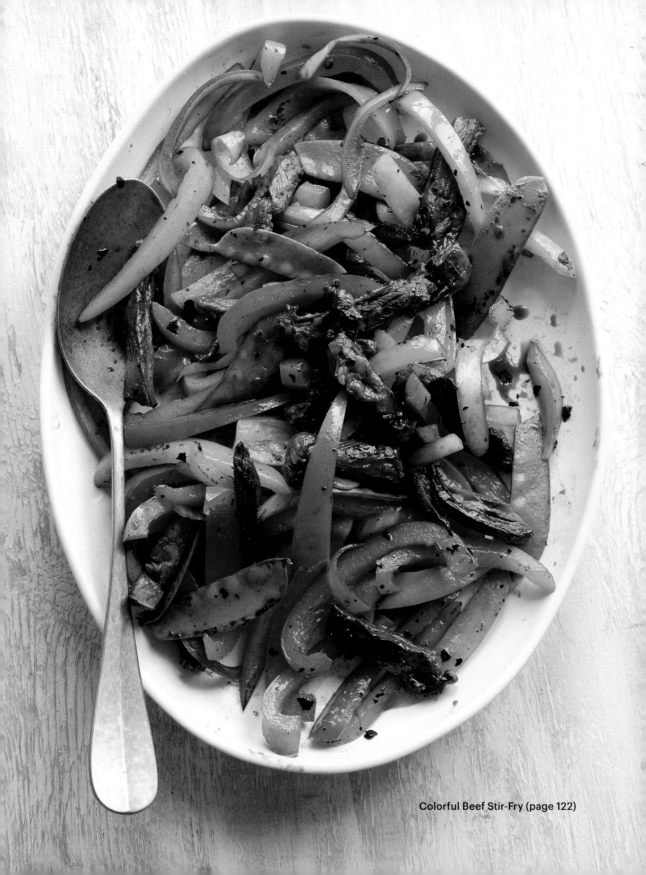

Colorful Beef Stir-Fry (page 122)

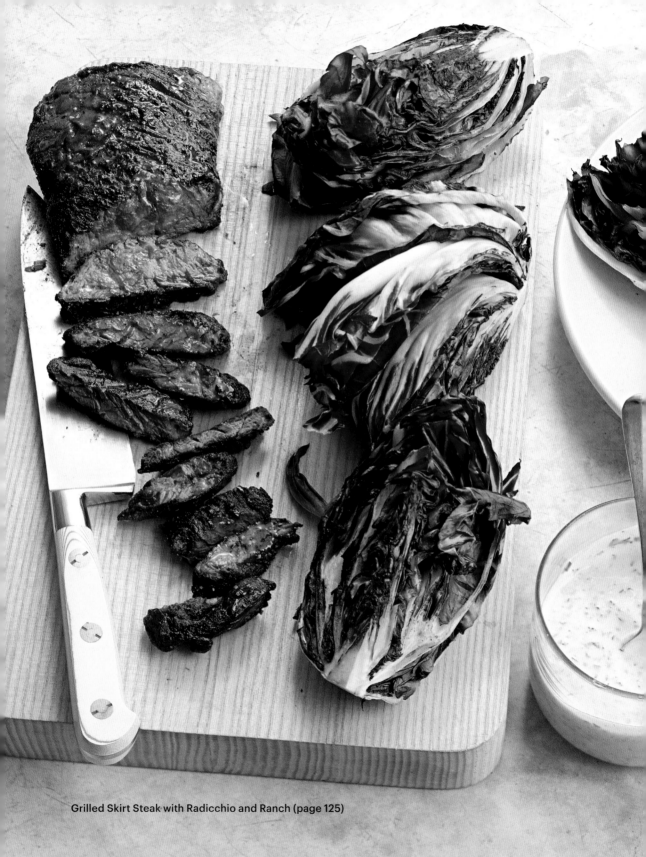

Grilled Skirt Steak with Radicchio and Ranch (page 125)

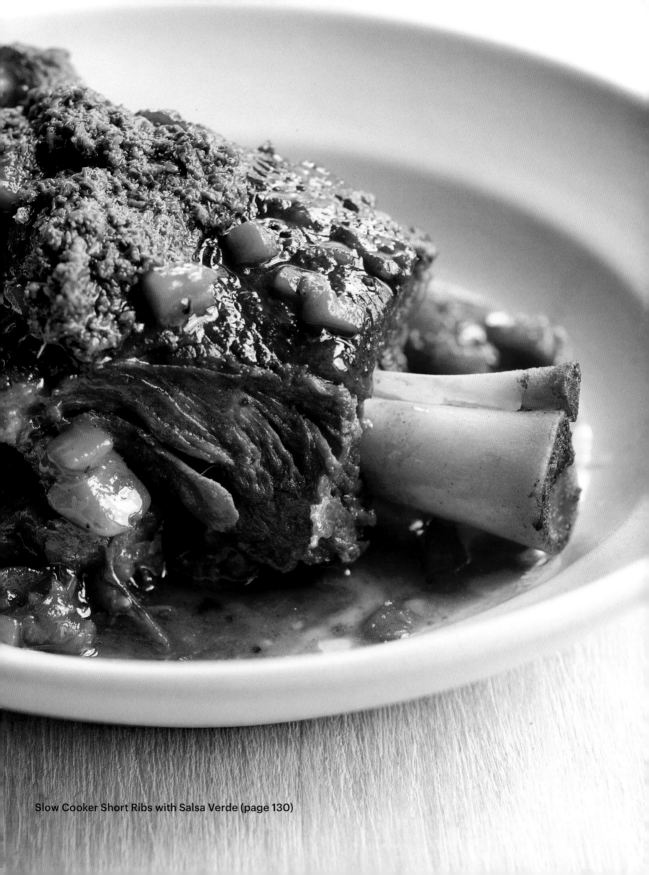

Slow Cooker Short Ribs with Salsa Verde (page 130)

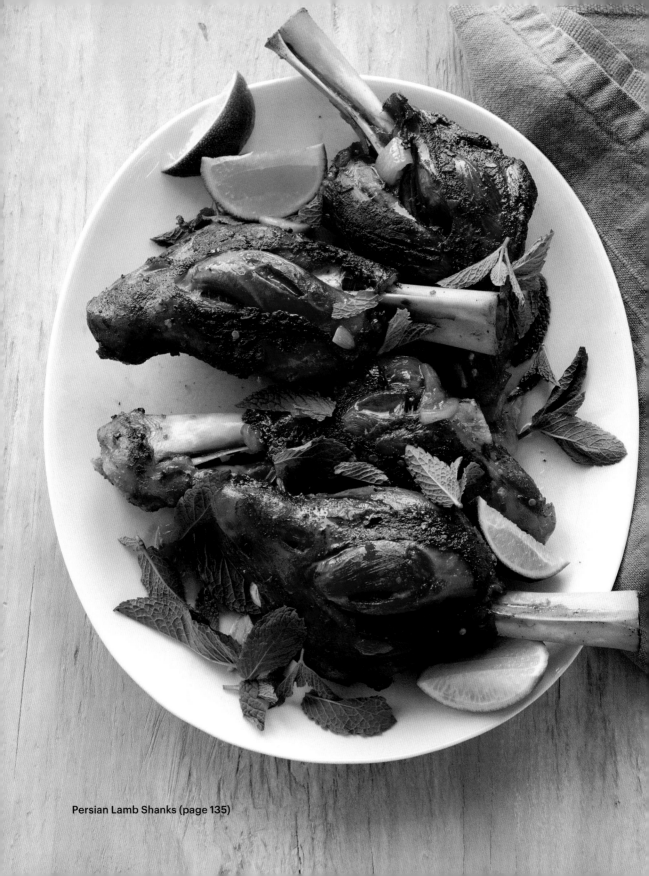

Persian Lamb Shanks (page 135)

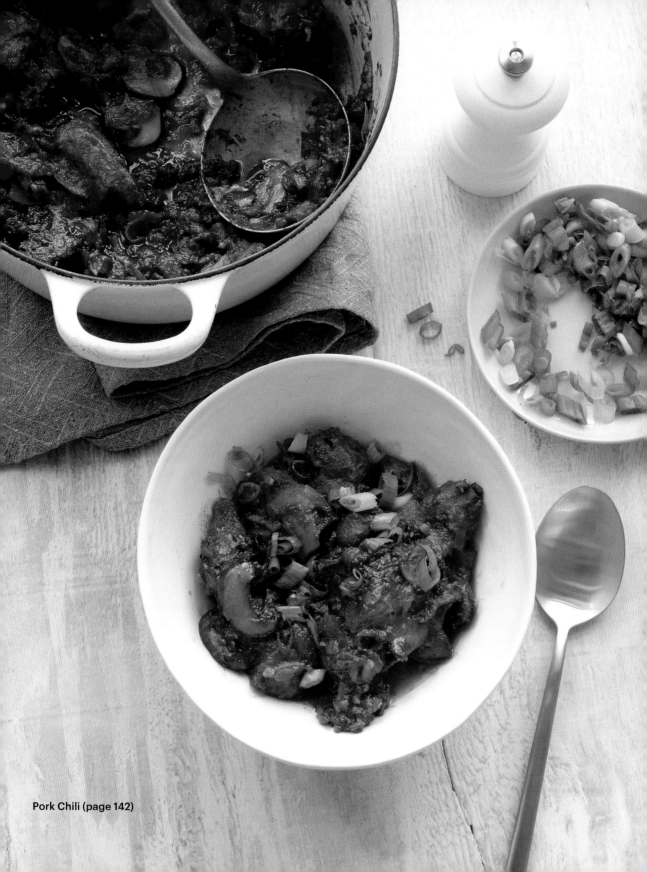

Pork Chili (page 142)

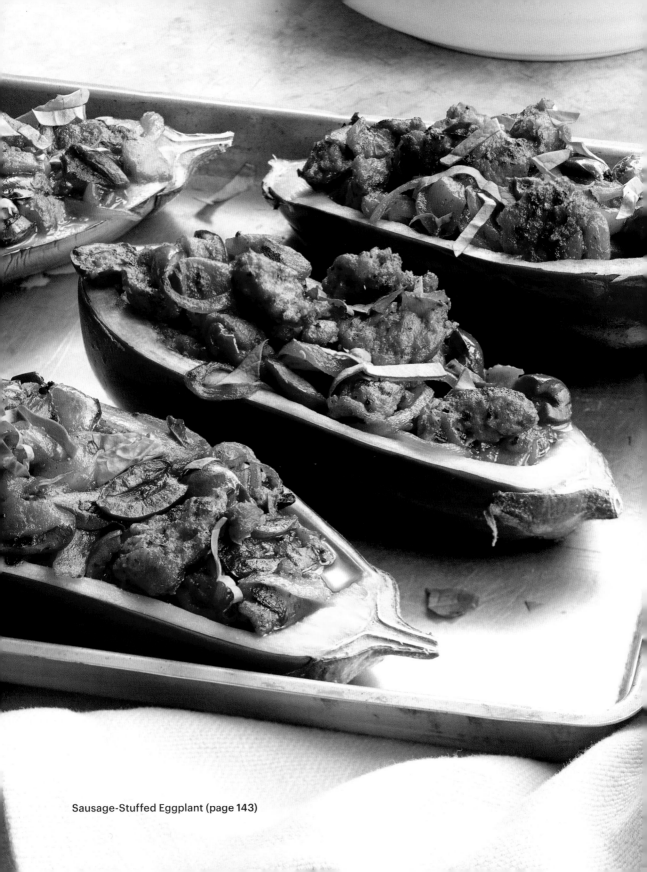

Sausage-Stuffed Eggplant (page 143)

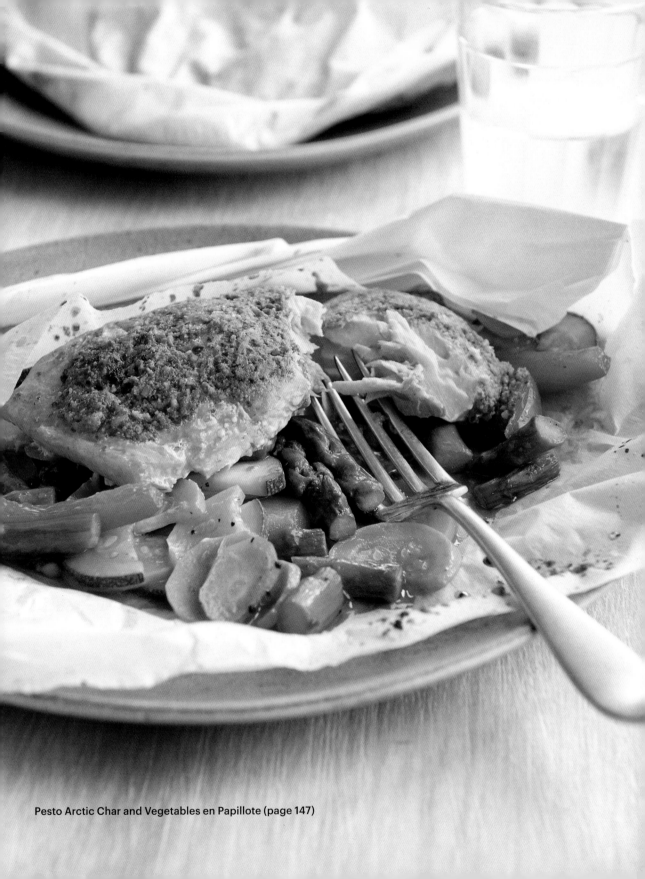

Pesto Arctic Char and Vegetables en Papillote (page 147)

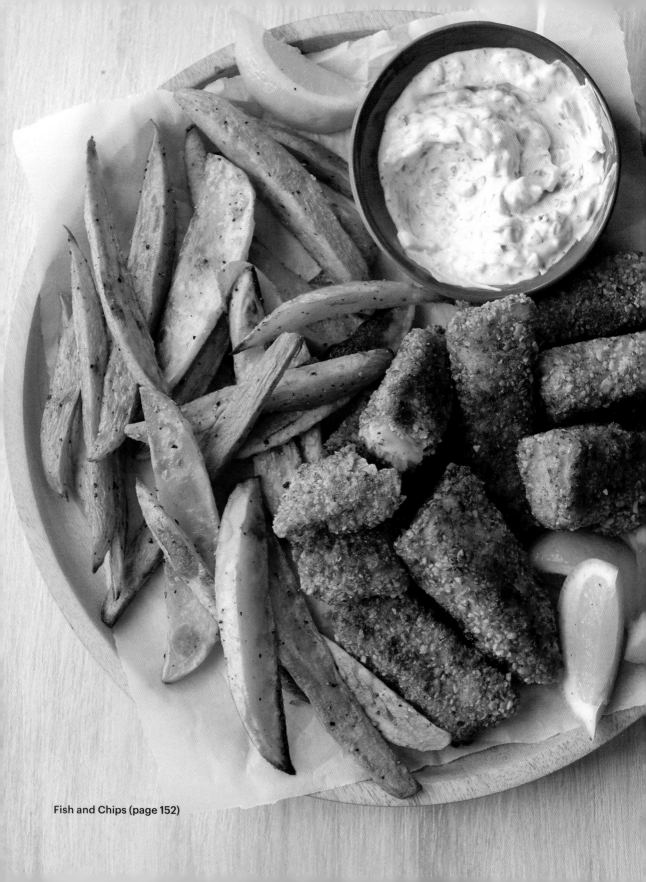

Fish and Chips (page 152)

# BACON-WRAPPED CHICKEN TENDERS

Both kids and adults love this super simple recipe, which I serve up with a side of avocado dipping sauce. Remember, be sure your bacon is sugar- and nitrate-free.

PREP TIME: 15 minutes

COOK TIME: 15 minutes

YIELD: 4 servings

PORTIONS: 1 protein, 1 fat

- 1 avocado, pitted and peeled
- 1 tablespoon olive oil
- ¼ cup chopped fresh cilantro
- ½ teaspoon Celtic or pink Himalayan salt
- ¼ teaspoon freshly ground black pepper
- 12 ounces chicken breast tenderloins
- 4 slices uncured bacon

Preheat the oven to 400°F.

In a small bowl, mash the avocado with the oil. Stir in the cilantro, salt, and pepper. Set aside.

Wrap each chicken tenderloin with ½ slice of bacon and place on a baking sheet. Bake until no longer pink and the juices run clear, 10 to 15 minutes, turning the tenders once (see Tip).

Serve with the avocado dipping sauce.

**TIP:** *If the bacon isn't crispy enough for you, put the baking sheet under the broiler for 1 to 2 minutes.*

# CHICKEN FRANCESE

Yes, you *can* have crispy pan-fried chicken on my diet! These coconut-crusted breast cutlets are fried to a golden brown, then simmered in a vibrant citrusy sauce.

PREP TIME: 10 minutes
COOK TIME: 15 minutes
YIELD: 4 servings
PORTIONS: 1 protein, 1 fat

⅓ cup coconut flour

½ teaspoon Celtic or pink Himalayan salt

½ teaspoon freshly ground black pepper

1 tablespoon cold ghee

1 egg, lightly beaten

Grated peel and juice of 1 lemon

4 chicken breast cutlets or thin-sliced breasts (about 1 pound)

¼ cup olive oil

¾ cup Chicken Bone Broth (page 65)

1½ tablespoons coarsely chopped fresh flat-leaf parsley or tarragon

Lemon wedges, for serving (optional)

In a shallow bowl or on a large plate, combine the flour with ¼ teaspoon each of the salt and pepper. Roll the ghee in the flour and set it aside. In another bowl or plate, combine the egg and lemon peel. Season the chicken with the remaining ¼ teaspoon each salt and pepper.

In a large pan, heat the oil over medium-high heat. Dredge the chicken completely in the flour, then in the egg, allowing excess egg to drip off. Add the chicken to the pan (in batches, if necessary) and cook until no longer pink and the juices run clear, about 4 minutes, turning once. Remove to a plate and pour out all but 2 tablespoons of the oil.

To the pan, add the broth and lemon juice, scraping the browned bits from the bottom of the pan, and cook for 2 minutes to reduce. Add the floured ghee and cook, stirring, until melted, 1 minute more. Add 1 tablespoon of the parsley and return the chicken to the skillet. Cook until heated through and the sauce thickens, about 3 minutes more.

Plate the chicken with a lemon wedge (if desired) and spoon the sauce over top. Sprinkle with the remaining parsley.

# CURRIED CASHEW CHICKEN

My quick curry sauce—a mix of cilantro, cashews, curry powder, and aromatic Asian-style bone broth—comes together in minutes in a food processor. This recipe calls for fresh chicken, but it's a terrific way to use leftover chicken as well.

PREP TIME: 10 minutes
COOK TIME: 20 minutes
YIELD: 4 servings
PORTIONS: 1 protein, 1 fat

- 1 cup packed cilantro leaves
- ½ cup raw cashews
- 1 tablespoon curry powder (see Tip)
- 1 clove garlic, peeled
- ½ teaspoon grated fresh ginger
- ¼ teaspoon Celtic or pink Himalayan salt
- 1 cup Asian Chicken Bone Broth (page 72)
- 1 pound boneless, skinless chicken thighs, cut into 1-inch pieces
- 1 red bell pepper, cut into ½-inch-wide strips
- 2 tablespoons fresh lime juice

In a food processor, combine the cilantro, ½ cup cashews, curry powder, garlic, ginger, and salt. Pulse until a paste forms. With the machine running, add the broth. The mixture will be thin and grainy. Transfer to a medium skillet and bring to a simmer over medium heat.

Tuck the chicken pieces into the sauce and simmer, stirring occasionally, until the chicken is no longer pink, about 12 minutes. Stir in the bell pepper and cook until just crisp-tender, about 3 minutes. Remove from the heat and stir in the lime juice.

TIP: *To kick up the heat, replace some (or all!) of the curry with hot Madras curry powder.*

## MAKE IT A 20

*Serve with quinoa: Cook 1 cup raw quinoa according to package directions in Asian Chicken Bone Broth instead of water.*

# TURKEY "POT PIE"

This healthy remake features a traditional pot pie filling, loaded with carrots, squash, leeks, green beans, and cubed turkey breast—all enveloped in silky, thickened turkey bone broth. Sprinkled with a nutty, streusel-like topping, it's a warming and filling any-night meal.

PREP TIME: 10 minutes

COOK TIME: 50 minutes

YIELD: 8 servings

PORTIONS: 1 protein, ½ fat, 1 vegetable, 1 starchy vegetable

1 tablespoon olive oil

1 large leek, white and light green parts, halved lengthwise and sliced crosswise into thin half-moons

2 carrots, finely chopped

2 cups Turkey Bone Broth (page 66)

½ pound peeled butternut squash, cut into ½-inch cubes (about ½ the base/bulb of 1 squash)

2 cups cooked and cubed turkey breast

1 cup frozen cut green beans

1 teaspoon Celtic or pink Himalayan salt

2 tablespoons arrowroot powder

3 tablespoons almond meal or ground almonds

2 tablespoons ground walnuts

2 tablespoons hulled pumpkin seeds

1 teaspoon minced fresh sage

1 teaspoon fresh thyme leaves

Coconut oil spray

Preheat the oven to 400°F.

In a large saucepan, heat the oil over medium heat. Add the leek and carrots and cook, stirring occasionally, until the leek is tender, about 6 minutes. Add the broth and squash and bring to a boil. Reduce the heat to low, cover, and simmer until the squash and carrots are tender, about 10 minutes. Stir in the turkey, green beans, and ½ teaspoon of the salt. Cook until heated through, about 2 minutes.

In a small bowl, stir together the arrowroot and 2 tablespoons water until smooth. Stir into the saucepan until well incorporated. Transfer the mixture to a 2-quart baking dish.

Toss together the almond meal, walnuts, pumpkin seeds, sage, thyme, and remaining ½ teaspoon salt. Sprinkle the mixture evenly over the filling in the baking dish, and then spray with coconut oil spray. Bake until the topping is golden and the filling is bubbling, 20 to 25 minutes. (Cover with foil if the top begins to brown too much.) Allow to sit for 10 minutes before serving.

## MAKE IT A 20

*Add ½ cup old-fashioned rolled oats to the food processor while making the topping, or serve the pot pie with brown rice noodles or quinoa.*

# CALIFORNIA PLATE with GREEN GODDESS DRESSING

Top deli turkey, hard-cooked eggs, grapes, artichoke hearts, sprouts, and cherry tomatoes with my fresh twist on a classic American salad dressing. This also makes a great layered salad in a Mason jar (see Tip).

PREP TIME: 15 minutes

YIELD: 4 servings

PORTIONS: 1 protein, 1 fat, 1 fruit

**For the dressing:**

- ¼ cup Homemade Mayonnaise (page 76)
- ¼ cup parsley leaves
- ¼ cup cilantro leaves
- 1 tablespoon finely chopped fresh chives
- 1 clove garlic, minced
- 1 teaspoon apple cider vinegar
- Celtic or pink Himalayan salt and freshly ground black pepper

**For the salad:**

- ½ pound deli-sliced turkey breast
- 4 large hard-cooked eggs, peeled and sliced
- 1 cup seedless green grapes
- 1 cup marinated artichoke hearts (from a 6-ounce jar)
- ½ cup alfalfa or radish sprouts
- 1 cup cherry tomatoes

*For the dressing:* In a food processor or blender, combine the mayonnaise, parsley, cilantro, chives, garlic, and vinegar. Process or blend until smooth, adding water, 1 tablespoon at a time, until desired consistency. Season to taste with salt and pepper.

*For the salad:* Divide the turkey, eggs, grapes, artichoke hearts, sprouts, and tomatoes among 4 plates and serve with the dressing drizzled over top or on the side.

**TIP:** *Make this a portable lunch by layering the ingredients in a large Mason jar, starting with the dressing at the bottom. When ready to eat, just shake it up!*

# MEDITERRANEAN PLATE
## with TAHINI DRESSING

Here's a quick and easy way to turn leftover chicken into a cool, light, and vibrant dish. Tahini gives the dressing a creamy, nutty flavor.

PREP TIME: 10 minutes

YIELD: 4 servings

PORTIONS: ½ protein, 1 fat, 1 vegetable

**For the dressing:**

- 2 tablespoons tahini
- 2 tablespoons olive oil
- 1 tablespoon fresh lemon juice
- ¼ teaspoon ground cumin
- ¼ teaspoon Celtic or pink Himalayan salt

**For the salad:**

- 2 cups shredded cooked chicken
- 1 medium cucumber, sliced into rounds
- 1 cup chopped tomato
- ½ cup jarred roasted red peppers, drained and cut into strips
- ½ cup sliced red onion

*For the dressing:* In a small bowl, stir together the tahini, oil, lemon juice, cumin, and salt until smooth.

*For the salad:* Divide the chicken, cucumber, tomatoes, roasted red peppers, and onions among 4 plates, and serve with the dressing drizzled over top or as a dip on the side.

# SPICY BRAISED CHICKEN THIGHS with FRIED CAPERS

Take everyday chicken to a new level! Capers add a salty bite, while star anise imparts a subtle licorice-like flavor.

PREP TIME: 15 minutes

COOK TIME: 40 minutes

YIELD: 4 servings

PORTIONS: 1 protein, 1 fat, 1 vegetable

- 2 tablespoons ghee
- 1 pound bone-in, skin-on chicken thighs
- Celtic or pink Himalayan salt and freshly ground black pepper
- 2 medium carrots, chopped
- 2 medium leeks, white and light green parts, halved lengthwise and sliced crosswise into half-moons
- 1 medium onion, chopped
- 4 cups Chicken Bone Broth (page 65)
- 3 cloves garlic, smashed
- 1 tablespoon black peppercorns
- 1 star anise
- 1 teaspoon crushed red-pepper flakes
- ¼ cup capers, drained
- 2 tablespoons olive oil

In a large skillet, heat the ghee over medium heat. Pat the chicken thighs dry with a paper towel and season with salt and pepper. Place the thighs in the skillet, skin side down, and sear until golden, about 2 minutes. Remove the chicken and set aside.

To the same skillet, add the carrots, leeks, and onion. Cook until softened, about 5 minutes.

Return the chicken to the pan and add the broth, garlic, peppercorns, star anise, and pepper flakes. Bring to a boil, then reduce the heat, cover, and simmer until a thermometer inserted in a chicken thigh registers 170°F and the vegetables are tender, about 25 minutes.

Meanwhile, pat the capers dry. In a small skillet, heat the oil over medium heat until shimmering. Add the capers and cook until crispy, about 2 minutes. Drain on paper towels.

Serve the chicken with some of the vegetables and topped with fried capers.

# SPICY TURKEY and BROCCOLI RABE

Fennel seeds and Italian seasoning give this easy meal a sophisticated flair. The leftovers are great in lettuce wraps.

PREP TIME: 5 minutes

COOK TIME: 15 minutes

YIELD: 4 servings

PORTIONS: 1 protein, ¼ fat, 1 vegetable

- 1 tablespoon olive oil
- 1 pound ground turkey
- 1 teaspoon Italian seasoning (see Tip)
- ¼ teaspoon fennel seeds
- 4 cloves garlic, sliced
- 1 bunch broccoli rabe, coarsely chopped
- 1 teaspoon crushed red-pepper flakes
- Celtic or pink Himalayan salt
- Lemon wedges, for serving

In a large skillet, heat the oil over medium heat. Add the turkey, Italian seasoning, and fennel seeds and cook, breaking it up with a wooden spoon, until the turkey is no longer pink, 4 to 5 minutes. Add the garlic and cook, stirring, for 1 minute. Add the broccoli rabe and cook until bright green and tender, about 5 minutes more. Stir in the pepper flakes, season to taste with salt, and serve with lemon wedges.

TIP: *Select Italian seasoning that is salt-, sugar-, dextrose-, and gluten-free.*

## MAKE IT A 20

*Serve tossed with rice-pasta shells or penne.*

# *Beef/Bison*

If you've been listening to those nutrition "experts" I've talked about, you may have a few qualms as you skim through the recipes in this section. That's because they contain red meat—and I know you've heard for years that the saturated fat in red meat is bad for your heart and your blood vessels.

Well, this is another myth that needs busting. In 2014, scientists reviewed 72 studies on the relationship between saturated fat and heart disease, involving more than 600,000 people. And you know what? The review found no link between either total dietary fat or saturated fat and heart disease.[1]

What's more, red meat is a wonderful source of nutrients that keep you healthy, including the omega-3s and conjugated linoleic acid (CLA) I talked about earlier. Pastured meat is particularly high in these nutrients.

So put my beef stir-fries, bison burgers, short ribs, and other tasty meat entrees on your menu. They taste fantastic, and they're very, very good for you!

# COLORFUL BEEF STIR-FRY

Break out the wok for this superfast dinner, and create a rainbow on your plate. Coconut aminos replace the soy sauce.

PREP TIME: 15 minutes
COOK TIME: 10 minutes

YIELD: 4 servings

PORTIONS: 1 protein, 1 fat, 1 vegetable

½ cup coconut aminos

¼ cup fresh orange juice

1 tablespoon toasted sesame oil

1 clove garlic, minced

1 small fresh red chile (optional), seeded and finely chopped (wear gloves when handling)

1 pound grass-fed flank steak, sliced into thin strips (see Tip)

2 tablespoons avocado oil

1 red bell pepper, sliced

1 yellow bell pepper, sliced

1 orange bell pepper, sliced

1 large onion, sliced

½ cup snow peas

1 teaspoon arrowroot powder

In a small bowl, stir together the coconut aminos, orange juice, sesame oil, garlic, and chile (if using). Measure out ½ cup and set aside. Place the sliced beef in a shallow dish and pour the remaining marinade mixture over it. Marinate for 15 minutes.

In a wok or large skillet, heat the avocado oil over medium-high heat. Remove the beef from the marinade (discard the marinade) and add to the wok. Cook until desired doneness, 1 to 2 minutes for medium. Remove the beef from the wok and set aside.

Add the bell peppers and onion to the wok and cook until crisp-tender, 1 to 2 minutes. Add the snow peas and cook until bright green, 1 minute more. Remove the vegetables from the wok. Add the reserved marinade and arrowroot powder to the wok and whisk to combine. Cook until the sauce is thickened and slightly reduced, 3 to 5 minutes. Return the beef and vegetables to the wok, toss to coat with the sauce, and serve.

TIP: For easy slicing, freeze the beef for 30 minutes beforehand.

## MAKE IT A 20

*Serve over your favorite brown rice noodles or brown basmati rice.*

# SLOW COOKER ROAST BEEF with SAUERKRAUT

Your slow cooker does nearly all the work here—just brown the meat and whip up a quick dressing. Caraway seeds add a distinctive Eastern European flavor to this dish.

PREP TIME: 15 minutes

COOK TIME: 6 to 8 hours

YIELD: 8 servings

PORTIONS: 1 protein, ½ fat

2 pounds beef tip roast, trimmed

Celtic or pink Himalayan salt and freshly ground black pepper

1 tablespoon olive oil

2 cups fermented sauerkraut, not drained (see Tip)

2 teaspoons caraway seeds

**For the Russian dressing:**

⅓ cup Homemade Mayonnaise (page 76)

3 tablespoons Homemade Ketchup (page 78)

1 tablespoon finely chopped onion

1 tablespoon chopped dill pickle

1 teaspoon fresh lemon juice

Pat the beef dry with paper towels and sprinkle with salt and pepper.

In a medium skillet, warm the oil over medium-high heat. Add the meat and brown on all sides, about 3 minutes per side.

Place the sauerkraut and caraway seeds in a slow cooker, along with the beef. Cover and cook on low until the meat is fork-tender, 6 to 8 hours.

*Meanwhile, make the Russian dressing*: In a bowl, stir together the mayonnaise, ketchup, onion, pickle, and lemon juice. Refrigerate until ready to serve.

Serve the beef with the sauerkraut and Russian dressing.

# CAVE MAN or WOMAN BURGERS

These juicy burgers get extra zip from balsamic vinaigrette. Add onions, mushrooms, and tomatoes for an all-American meal.

PREP TIME: 10 minutes

COOK TIME: 50 minutes

YIELD: 4 servings

PORTIONS: 1 protein, ½ fat, 1 vegetable

1 pound ground bison

2 tablespoons Balsamic Vinaigrette (page 80)

Celtic or pink Himalayan salt and freshly ground black pepper

2 tablespoons olive oil

2 medium yellow onions, thinly sliced

1 pound wild mushrooms, sliced

1 large heirloom tomato, cut into 4 thick slices

1 cup baby arugula

In a bowl, combine the bison, vinaigrette, ½ teaspoon salt, and ½ teaspoon pepper and mix well. Form into four ¾-inch-thick patties, cover, and refrigerate until ready to cook.

In a large skillet, heat 1 tablespoon of the oil over medium-high heat until shimmering. Add the onions, mushrooms, and a large pinch of salt and cook, stirring frequently, until completely wilted and beginning to stick to the bottom of the pan, about 10 minutes. Reduce the heat to low and cook, stirring and scraping the pan with a wooden spoon every few minutes. If the mixture looks like it's burning, add a couple tablespoons of water and stir. Continue cooking until the onions and mushrooms are a uniform caramel brown, 30 to 45 minutes more. Add another couple tablespoons of water, stir, and scrape up the bottom of the pan. Use right away or let cool to room temperature and store in an airtight container in the refrigerator for up to 1 week or in the freezer for up to 1 month.

When ready to serve, heat the remaining 1 tablespoon oil over medium heat. Add the burgers to the skillet and cook, turning once, until a thermometer inserted in the center of a burger registers 160°F and the meat is no longer pink, about 10 minutes.

Serve the burgers on top of the tomato slices with arugula and a big spoonful of caramelized onions and mushrooms.

# GRILLED SKIRT STEAK with RADICCHIO and RANCH

This simple salt-and-pepper steak is grilled medium-rare, thinly sliced, and served on a bed of grilled radicchio topped with ranch dressing. In addition to adding flavor, marinating tenderizes the meat.

PREP TIME: 5 minutes
COOK TIME: 1 hour 15 minutes (mostly unattended)
YIELD: 4 servings
PORTIONS: 1 protein, 1 fat

1 pound beef skirt steak, cut into 4 portions

½ cup My Favorite Marinade (page 81)

1 head radicchio, quartered

¼ cup Ranch Dressing (page 84)

In a large zip-top plastic bag, combine the steak and marinade and marinate for 1 hour at room temperature or overnight in the refrigerator.

Preheat a gas grill or grill pan to medium heat. Remove the steak from the marinade (discard the marinade) and grill for about 4 minutes per side (or until desired doneness). At the same time, grill the radicchio until slightly wilted, about 5 minutes, turning to grill both cut sides.

Let the steak rest for 10 minutes before thinly slicing against the grain. Serve with a radicchio wedge drizzled with ranch dressing.

# VIETNAMESE BEEF SALAD

From rice vinegar and fish sauce to basil, mint, ginger, and sesame, the flavors of Vietnam make this dish sing. Turn leftovers into lettuce wraps for lunch the next day!

PREP TIME: 10 minutes
COOK TIME: 25 minutes

YIELD: 2 servings

PORTIONS: 1 protein, 1 fat, 1 vegetable

1 tablespoon rice vinegar

1 teaspoon fish sauce

1 tablespoon plus 1 teaspoon olive oil

½ napa cabbage, shredded

2 medium carrots, shredded

1 tablespoon chopped basil leaves, plus more for garnish

1 tablespoon chopped mint leaves, plus more for garnish

1 clove garlic, minced

1 teaspoon minced fresh ginger

½ pound ground beef

1 teaspoon toasted sesame oil

Celtic or pink Himalayan salt and freshly ground black pepper

1 small head butter lettuce, leaves separated

2 or 3 radishes, thinly sliced

¼ cup bean sprouts

In a medium bowl, whisk together the rice vinegar, fish sauce, and 1 tablespoon of the olive oil. Add the cabbage, carrots, basil, and mint and toss to combine. Let the slaw rest at room temperature to meld the flavors while you cook the beef.

In a skillet, heat the remaining 1 teaspoon olive oil over medium heat. Add the garlic and ginger and cook for 1 minute. Add the ground beef and cook, breaking it up with a spoon, until no longer pink, about 5 minutes. Remove from the heat, drain off any excess fat, drizzle with the sesame oil, and season to taste with salt and pepper.

To assemble, place a few lettuce leaves on each of 2 plates and arrange the slaw, beef, sliced radishes, and sprouts on top. Sprinkle with the basil and mint.

## MAKE IT A 20

*Add 1 cup cooked rice noodles underneath the beef.*

# STUFFED PEPPERS

Cumin, coriander, and the smoky flavor of chipotle give these veggie-loaded peppers a hint of heat. Top with cilantro for extra Mexican flavor.

PREP TIME: 15 minutes

COOK TIME: 25 minutes

YIELD: 4 servings

PORTIONS: 1 protein, ½ fat, 2 vegetable

- 2 tablespoons olive oil
- 1 pound ground bison or lean ground beef
- 4 bell peppers (any color), tops cut off and chopped, cores removed
- 1 pint cherry or grape tomatoes, halved
- 1 yellow onion, finely chopped
- 1 zucchini, cut into ½-inch cubes
- 1 Chipotle in Adobo (optional; page 87), finely chopped
- 2 cloves garlic, minced
- 1 teaspoon ground cumin
- 1 teaspoon ground coriander
- ¼ teaspoon Celtic or pink Himalayan salt
- ¼ teaspoon freshly ground black pepper
- Chopped fresh cilantro, for garnish

Preheat the oven to 375°F.

In a large skillet, heat 2 teaspoons of the oil over medium heat. Add the bison or beef and cook, stirring occasionally and breaking it up with a spoon until no longer pink, about 5 minutes.

If the skillet seems dry, add the remaining 1 tablespoon oil. Add the chopped pepper tops, tomatoes, onion, zucchini, chipotle (if using), garlic, cumin, coriander, salt, and pepper. Cook, stirring occasionally, until the bell peppers and onion are soft and the tomatoes have cooked down, about 8 minutes.

Meanwhile, place the bell peppers in an ovenproof 9-inch pie plate or 8 × 8-inch baking dish. (If the peppers don't stand up, carefully shave a bit off the bottoms, without cutting through, so that they're level.)

Divide the meat mixture among the peppers. Pour ½ cup water in the bottom of the dish, cover, and bake until the peppers are softened and the tops are browned, about 30 minutes. Serve sprinkled with cilantro.

## MAKE IT A 20

*Cook 1 cup quinoa according to package directions using Beef Bone Broth (page 67) instead of water. Mix the cooked quinoa into the stuffing.*

# NOT-YOUR-MOTHER'S MEATLOAF with TURNIP MASH

Gourmet meatloaf? You bet! My version features cremini mushrooms, sherry vinegar, and both beef and bison. A side of buttery turnip mash rounds out the plate.

PREP TIME: 20 minutes
COOK TIME: 1 hour 10 minutes

YIELD: 6 servings

PORTIONS: 1 protein, 1 fat, 1 vegetable

## For the meatloaf:

- 1 tablespoon olive oil
- 8 ounces cremini (baby bella) mushrooms, finely chopped
- ½ medium yellow onion, finely chopped
- 1 medium carrot, finely chopped
- 1 clove garlic, minced
- 2 tablespoons sherry vinegar
- ¾ pound ground beef
- ¾ pound ground bison
- 2 tablespoons almond meal
- 2 large eggs, beaten
- ¼ cup chopped fresh flat-leaf parsley
- ½ teaspoon dry mustard
- Celtic or pink Himalayan salt and freshly ground black pepper
- ¼ cup Homemade Ketchup (page 78)

*For the meatloaf:* In a large skillet, heat the oil over medium heat. Add the mushrooms, onion, carrot, and garlic and cook until all the vegetables are softened and beginning to brown, about 10 minutes. Add the sherry vinegar and cook until the skillet is almost dry, about 2 minutes. Transfer to a large bowl and let cool to room temperature.

Position a rack in the center of the oven and preheat to 375°F. Line a large rimmed baking sheet with parchment or foil.

To the bowl of cooled vegetables, add the beef, bison, almond meal, eggs, parsley, mustard, 1 teaspoon salt, and ½ teaspoon pepper. Using your hands, mix gently to combine. Transfer the meatloaf mixture to the prepared baking sheet. Form into a rectangular loaf about 6 × 3 inches. Brush the ketchup all over the surface of the meatloaf and bake until a thermometer inserted in the center registers 160°F and the meat is no longer pink, 35 to 45 minutes. Let rest for 10 minutes before slicing.

## For the turnips:

- 1 large rutabaga (yellow turnip), about 2 pounds, peeled and cut into 1-inch chunks
- Celtic or pink Himalayan salt
- ½ cup canned coconut milk, well stirred
- 2 tablespoons ghee
- Freshly ground black pepper
- ¼ cup sliced fresh chives

*For the turnips:* Place the turnip chunks in a saucepan with water to cover and a pinch of salt. Bring to a boil, then reduce the heat and simmer, partly covered, until easily pierced with a fork, about 20 minutes. Drain.

Puree the turnips in a food processor until smooth. Pulse in the coconut milk and ghee and season to taste with salt and pepper. Sprinkle with chives and serve alongside the meatloaf.

# SLOW COOKER SHORT RIBS with SALSA VERDE

These ribs are so tender, you can eat them with a spoon. Top with a dollop of salsa to add a little zest.

PREP TIME: 10 minutes

COOK TIME: 5 to 8 hours (depending on the slow cooker setting)

YIELD: 8 servings

PORTIONS: 1 protein, 1 fat

**For the short ribs:**

- 2 tablespoons extra-virgin olive oil
- 4 large beef short ribs (14–16 ounces each)
- Celtic or pink Himalayan salt and freshly ground black pepper
- 6 cups Italian Beef Bone Broth (page 75)
- 1 small yellow onion, finely chopped
- 1 small carrot, finely chopped
- 1 small rib celery, finely chopped
- 2 tablespoons balsamic vinegar
- 2 sprigs thyme
- 1 bay leaf

*For the short ribs:* In a large skillet, heat the oil over medium-high heat. Season the short ribs generously with salt and pepper. Add the short ribs to the pan and sear each side until a golden brown crust forms, about 7 minutes per side. Transfer the short ribs to a 6-quart slow cooker. Add the broth, onion, carrot, celery, vinegar, thyme, and bay leaf. Cover and cook until the meat is fork-tender, about 4 hours on high or 7 hours on low. Transfer the short ribs to a serving platter and cover with foil to rest for 30 minutes.

## For the salsa verde:

- 1 tablespoon capers, rinsed and drained
- 1 small clove garlic, chopped
- 1 anchovy fillet (preferably salt-packed), rinsed
- 1 cup loosely packed flat-leaf parsley leaves
- ¼ cup loosely packed mint leaves
- 1 teaspoon chopped fresh oregano
- ⅓ cup extra-virgin olive oil

*For the salsa verde:* While the short ribs are resting, in a food processor, combine the capers, garlic, and anchovy and pulse until finely chopped. Add the parsley, mint, and oregano and pulse until finely chopped and completely combined. Transfer the mixture to a medium bowl and stir in the oil.

Strain the liquid from the slow cooker through a fine-mesh sieve into a saucepan. Skim off the fat and bring the liquid to a boil over high heat. Cook until reduced by half and slightly thickened, about 15 minutes.

Divide the short ribs among 4 bowls. Drizzle with the reduced braising liquid and the salsa verde.

# BROILED CHIPOTLE FLANK STEAK with ROASTED SWEET POTATOES and ONIONS

Roasting brings out the rich, sweet flavors of the sweet potatoes and onions, which pair beautifully with the spicy seasoned steak. This entire meal cooks on one foil-lined baking sheet, for easy cleanup.

PREP TIME: 10 minutes
COOK TIME: 25 minutes

YIELD: 4 servings

PORTIONS: 1 protein, ¼ fat, 1 starchy vegetable

2 large sweet potatoes, peeled and cut into 1-inch chunks

1 cup frozen pearl onions, thawed

1 tablespoon olive oil

Celtic or pink Himalayan salt and freshly ground black pepper

2 tablespoons minced Chipotles in Adobo (page 87)

1 tablespoon fresh lime juice

½ teaspoon ground cumin

1 pound flank steak

Position a rack 6 inches below the broiler and preheat the oven to 425°F. Line a large rimmed baking sheet with foil.

Toss the sweet potatoes and onions with 2 teaspoons of the oil and salt and pepper. Spread on the prepared sheet. Roast until the potatoes begin to soften and color slightly, about 12 minutes.

Meanwhile, in a small bowl, combine the chipotles, lime juice, and cumin.

Turn the broiler on high. Rub the remaining 1 teaspoon oil over the steak and season with salt. Turn the sweet potatoes and onions, push them to one side of the sheet, and place the steak on the other half. Broil until the steak is browned, about 3 minutes.

Remove the steak from the oven, turn over, and spread the chipotle mixture over the steak. If the vegetables are tender, transfer them to a serving plate. Return the steak to the oven and broil until desired doneness, about 4 minutes more for medium-rare. (At medium-rare, a thermometer inserted in the center will register 145°F.) Transfer to a cutting board and let rest for 5 minutes before slicing against the grain.

Serve the steak slices with the roasted vegetables.

# PAN-ROASTED LIVER and ONIONS with MUSTARD SAUCE

How do you make liver and onions taste heavenly? By caramelizing the onions in bacon drippings, giving the liver a quick sear until it's barely pink inside, and topping everything off with a velvety sauce.

PREP TIME: 10 minutes
COOK TIME: 45 minutes
YIELD: 4 servings
PORTIONS: 1 protein, ¼ fat

4 slices uncured bacon

2 Vidalia or other sweet onions, sliced

½ teaspoon Celtic or pink Himalayan salt

1 tablespoon olive oil, if needed

12 ounces calf's or veal liver (see Tip), cut crosswise into 1-inch-thick slices

2 tablespoons red wine vinegar

½ cup Beef Bone Broth (page 67) or French Onion Beef Bone Broth (page 74)

2 tablespoons whole-grain Dijon mustard

¼ cup fresh flat-leaf parsley, coarsely chopped

In a large skillet, cook the bacon over medium heat until crisp, about 8 minutes. Remove the bacon to a plate lined with paper towels and crumble when cool.

To the skillet, add the onions and salt. Cook, stirring occasionally, until deeply golden and very soft, 20 to 25 minutes.

Transfer the onions to a serving plate and cover with foil to keep warm. If the skillet seems dry, add the oil and return to medium heat. When hot, add the liver. Sear for 3 to 4 minutes, turn, and sear until desired doneness, 3 to 5 minutes more. Remove the liver to the serving plate and cover.

Add the vinegar to the skillet and allow to nearly evaporate. Add the broth and bring to a simmer, scraping up the browned bits from the bottom of the skillet. Cook until reduced by half, about 5 minutes. Add the mustard and stir until combined. Stir in the parsley and reserved crumbled bacon.

To serve, pour the sauce over the liver and onions.

TIP: *Liver is sold in many forms, from a 1-pound slab to thin strips resembling bacon. However your liver is sold, the key is to sear it on both sides until browned, cooking until the center is just barely pink.*

## MAKE IT A 20

*Serve with cottage potatoes (thick-cut, peeled potatoes, pan-fried until golden).*

# *Pork/Lamb*

I always say, "Don't sweat it if you can't afford organic or pastured meat." However, there's one meat I'd like you to try to buy organic or pastured whenever possible, or otherwise use somewhat sparingly: pork. There's a huge difference in quality between factory-farmed and pastured pork, so it's worth spending a little extra money if you can find it in your budget.

Lamb is a great choice for meals because you can always find grass-fed cuts, and lamb chops cook quickly when you're in a hurry. (For instance, try my Thai-Spiced Lamb Chops—delicious, and done in minutes.) Lamb is a little pricey, but if you buy it in bulk at a "big box" store, you can get a good deal. Ground lamb, in particular, is pretty cheap—and when you use it in recipes like my Lamb Koftas with Lemon-Tahini Sauce, it tastes like a million bucks!

# PERSIAN LAMB SHANKS

Aromatic spices—turmeric, cinnamon, and cardamom—turn simple lamb shanks into an exotic dish. Fresh mint and lime wedges are traditional accents.

PREP TIME: 10 minutes
COOK TIME: 1 hour 30 minutes
YIELD: 4 servings
PORTIONS: 1 protein, ½ fat

- 1 teaspoon crushed red-pepper flakes
- 1 teaspoon Celtic or pink Himalayan salt
- 1 teaspoon freshly ground black pepper
- ½ teaspoon ground turmeric
- ½ teaspoon ground cinnamon
- ¼ teaspoon ground cardamom
- 4 meaty lamb shanks
- 2 tablespoons olive oil
- 1 medium onion, cut into wedges
- 4 cloves garlic, halved
- 3 cups Beef Bone Broth (page 67)
- ¼ cup mint leaves, for serving
- Lime wedges, for serving

Preheat the oven to 400°F.

In a small bowl, stir together the pepper flakes, salt, pepper, turmeric, cinnamon, and cardamom. Rub all over the lamb shanks.

In a roasting pan, heat the oil over medium-high heat. Add the lamb shanks and cook, turning, until browned on all sides, about 5 minutes total. Remove the shanks from the pan and add the onion and garlic. Cook until softened, about 5 minutes. Add the broth and return the shanks to the pan. Bring to a boil, then cover tightly with foil and place in the oven.

Bake until the lamb is tender and falling off the bone, 1 hour to 1 hour 30 minutes. Serve garnished with mint leaves and lime wedges.

# PORK RAGU with ZUCCHINI PAPPARDELLE

When you grow up in an Italian household, there's always a pot of sauce simmering on the stove. This ragu, served with zucchini "pasta," transports me right back to my childhood.

PREP TIME: 10 minutes
COOK TIME: 1 hour 30 minutes

YIELD: 4 servings

PORTIONS: 1 protein, ½ fat, 1 vegetable

1 ounce dried porcini mushrooms

1 cup boiling water

2 tablespoons ghee

1 medium yellow onion, finely chopped

2 medium carrots, finely chopped

1 medium rib celery, finely chopped

Celtic or pink Himalayan salt and freshly ground black pepper

3 tablespoons tomato paste

1 pound ground pork

½ cup red wine*

1½ cups Beef Bone Broth (page 67) or water

½ teaspoon ground nutmeg

2 large zucchini, washed and trimmed

In a small heatproof bowl, soak the porcinis in the boiling water for 15 minutes. Scoop out the mushrooms and chop. Strain and reserve the soaking liquid.

In a large, heavy pot or Dutch oven, heat the ghee over medium-high heat. Add the onion, carrots, celery, and a pinch of salt and pepper and cook, stirring, until the vegetables soften, about 8 minutes. Add the porcinis and tomato paste and cook until the paste darkens a shade, about 4 minutes more.

Add the pork and cook, breaking it up with a wooden spoon, until just browned, about 5 minutes. Add the wine and let reduce by half, about 5 minutes more. Add the broth and reserved mushroom soaking liquid, reduce the heat to low, partially cover, and simmer until the liquid is mostly absorbed but there is still movement to the sauce, about 1 hour. Stir in the nutmeg and a generous amount of pepper.

Meanwhile, using a vegetable peeler, peel the zucchini into 1-inch-wide "noodles," like pappardelle pasta. Bring a large pot of well-salted water to a boil and blanch the zucchini until just tender, about 1 minute. Drain.

In a large bowl, toss the zucchini noodles with about 1 cup ragu to coat. Divide among 4 plates and top with additional ragu.

## MAKE IT A 20

*Serve with your favorite brown rice or ancient-grain pasta instead of the zucchini.*

*\*Wine is allowed on the basic Bone Broth Diet if the alcohol is cooked off.*

# OVEN-BAKED PORK CHOPS with SAUERKRAUT and APPLES

In this old-fashioned, country-style dish, bone-in pork chops roast with apple wedges. Serve on a bed of gently heated sauerkraut for a delicious mix of sweet and tangy flavors.

PREP TIME: 5 minutes
COOK TIME: 20 minutes
YIELD: 4 servings
PORTIONS: 1 protein, ¼ fat, 1 fruit

- 4 bone-in pork chops (about 1-inch thick)
- 1 tablespoon olive oil
- ½ teaspoon Celtic or pink Himalayan salt
- ½ teaspoon freshly ground black pepper
- ½ teaspoon dried thyme
- ¼ teaspoon ground sage
- 2 apples, each cored and cut into 8 wedges
- 2 cups fermented sauerkraut, drained

About 30 minutes before cooking, take the pork chops out of the refrigerator. Preheat the oven to 400°F.

Heat a large ovenproof skillet over medium-high heat. Rub the pork chops with the oil and sprinkle with salt, pepper, thyme, and sage. Set the chops in the hot skillet and sear until a dark golden crust forms, about 3 minutes. Use tongs to turn the chops. Scatter the apples around the pork and transfer the skillet to the oven. Roast until a thermometer inserted in the center of a chop registers 160°F, 6 to 8 minutes.

Remove the skillet from the oven. Transfer the pork to a plate and cover with foil to keep warm.

To the skillet, add the sauerkraut, stirring to combine with the pan drippings and apples. Cook until heated through, 3 to 4 minutes.

To serve, divide the sauerkraut and apples among 4 plates and top each with a pork chop.

### MAKE IT A 20

*Put peeled and sliced potatoes in the oven as soon as it reaches 400°F.*

# PORK and VEGETABLE ADOBO

*Adobo* is a Spanish word for sauce or marinade. This recipe features classic adobo ingredients including garlic and vinegar, along with coconut aminos to give the dish depth and a rich brown color.

PREP TIME: 10 minutes

COOK TIME: 20 minutes

YIELD: 4 servings

PORTIONS: 1 protein, ¼ fat, 1 vegetable

---

- 1 tablespoon avocado oil
- 1 pound pork tenderloin, trimmed and cut into strips
- Celtic or pink Himalayan salt and freshly ground black pepper
- 4 large cloves garlic, minced
- ¼ cup distilled white vinegar
- ¼ cup coconut aminos
- 1 bay leaf
- ½ teaspoon freshly cracked black peppercorns
- 2 cups steamed broccoli florets
- 2 cups trimmed sugar snap peas, halved
- 1 cup steamed carrot slices

In a heavy-duty 12-inch skillet, heat the oil over medium-high heat. Add the pork, season with a pinch of salt and ground pepper and cook, stirring occasionally, until light golden brown, 4 to 6 minutes. Add the garlic and cook, stirring occasionally, for 2 minutes more. Add the vinegar, coconut aminos, bay leaf, and cracked pepper. Bring to a boil, reduce the heat to medium-low, and simmer until the liquid reduces by about one-quarter, 6 to 8 minutes. Discard the bay leaf.

Toss in the broccoli, sugar snap peas, and carrots and cook for about 2 minutes to warm through.

## MAKE IT A 20

*Serve over brown basmati rice to soak up all the sauce.*

# CUBAN PULLED PORK

Succulent pork blends with onion, garlic, and three citrus juices to create a roast so tender you can shred it. Simply pop your ingredients into a slow cooker for an effortless meal.

**PREP TIME:** 10 minutes
**COOK TIME:** 3 to 5 hours (depending on the slow cooker setting)
**YIELD:** 8 servings
**PORTIONS:** 1 protein, ¼ fat

- 1 small white onion, thinly sliced
- 2 pounds boneless, skinless pork shoulder
- ¼ cup fresh orange juice
- 2 tablespoons extra-virgin olive oil
- 2 tablespoons fresh lemon juice
- 2 tablespoons fresh lime juice
- 6 cloves garlic, minced
- 1 teaspoon Celtic or pink Himalayan salt
- 1 teaspoon dried oregano
- 1 teaspoon coarsely ground black pepper

Scatter the onion over the bottom of a 6-quart slow cooker and place the pork on top. Using a sharp paring knife, poke holes all over the entire pork shoulder.

In a small bowl, combine the orange juice, oil, lemon juice, lime juice, garlic, salt, oregano, and pepper and pour over the pork. Using your fingers, poke some of the sauce into the holes. Cover and cook until the meat falls apart, about 3 hours on high, or 5 hours on low.

Shred the meat using 2 forks and toss with the sauce in the slow cooker.

## MAKE IT A 20

*Serve with black beans and a salad.*

# LAMB KOFTAS with LEMON-TAHINI SAUCE

Everybody loves meat on a stick! In this recipe, a light, lemony drizzle sauce balances out the richness of the lamb.

PREP TIME: 10 minutes

COOK TIME: 40 minutes plus 1 to 5 hours sitting time

YIELD: 4 servings

PORTIONS: 1 protein, ½ fat

### For the koftas:

- 8 flat, wide wooden skewers (12 inches)
- 1 pound ground lamb
- ½ medium red onion, grated
- 1 clove garlic, minced
- 1 teaspoon ground cumin
- ¾ teaspoon Celtic or pink Himalayan salt
- ½ teaspoon ground coriander
- ½ teaspoon cracked black pepper
- ¼ teaspoon ground cinnamon
- Pinch of ground allspice

*For the koftas:* In a 13 × 9-inch baking dish, soak the skewers in warm water for 30 minutes.

In a large bowl, using your hands, mix together the lamb, onion, garlic, cumin, salt, coriander, pepper, cinnamon, and allspice until combined and the meat is a bit sticky. With wet hands, divide the lamb into 8 equal portions.

Working with one portion at a time (rewetting your hands as necessary to prevent sticking), press the lamb around the skewers into 4½-inch-long sausage shapes. Place on a platter or cutting board, cover loosely with plastic wrap, and refrigerate for at least 1 hour and up to 5 hours.

Preheat a gas or charcoal grill to medium-high heat. Oil the grates with olive or avocado oil. Grill the skewers, turning every 2 minutes, until grill marks form all over and the meat is no longer pink in the center, about 8 minutes.

## For the sauce:

- 2 tablespoons tahini
- 1 tablespoon extra-virgin olive oil
- 1 tablespoon finely chopped fresh flat-leaf parsley
- 2 teaspoons fresh lemon juice, plus more to taste
- 1 small clove garlic, minced
- Celtic or pink Himalayan salt
- Cayenne pepper

*For the sauce:* In a large bowl, whisk together the tahini, olive oil, parsley, lemon juice, garlic, and 2 tablespoons water until smooth. Season to taste with salt, cayenne, and additional lemon juice.

To serve, drizzle the sauce over the skewers.

# PORK CHILI

I take this chili to tailgate parties, and there's never a bite left over. The pork is an interesting change of pace from the usual hamburger.

PREP TIME: 15 minutes

COOK TIME: 45 minutes

YIELD: 4 servings

PORTIONS: 1 protein, negligible fat, 1 vegetable

- 1 tablespoon olive oil
- 1 pound pork tenderloin, cubed
- 1 teaspoon Celtic or pink Himalayan salt, plus more to taste
- ½ teaspoon freshly ground black pepper, plus more to taste
- 1 medium onion, chopped
- 2 cloves garlic, minced
- 1 green bell pepper, chopped
- 4 ounces mixed mushrooms, sliced
- 1 jalapeño pepper (optional), seeded and finely chopped (wear gloves when handling)
- 1 can (28 ounces) crushed tomatoes
- 1 cup Beef Bone Broth (page 67)
- 1 teaspoon ground cumin
- ½ teaspoon dried oregano
- 2 or 3 scallions, thinly sliced

In a large pot, heat the oil over medium heat. Season the pork with salt and pepper, add to the pot, and brown on all sides, about 2 minutes per side. Remove the meat from the pot.

Add the onion and garlic to the pot and cook until softened, about 4 minutes. Add the bell pepper, mushrooms, and jalapeño (if using) and cook until beginning to soften, 3 minutes more. Return the meat to the pot and add the tomatoes, broth, cumin, and oregano and bring to a boil. Reduce the heat and simmer until thickened, about 30 minutes. Season to taste with salt and pepper.

Serve topped with scallions.

# SAUSAGE-STUFFED EGGPLANT

Savory Italian sausage and mild, mellow eggplant were simply made for each other. I prefer using smaller Japanese egg-plants, so everyone has their own eggplant "bowl."

PREP TIME: 10 minutes

COOK TIME: 45 minutes

YIELD: 4 servings

PORTIONS: ½ protein, ¼ fat, 1 vegetable

½ pound Italian sausage (casings removed if in links)

4 Japanese eggplants or 2 medium eggplants, halved lengthwise

4 teaspoons olive oil

1 tomato, chopped

⅓ cup black olives, pitted and chopped

¼ white onion, thinly sliced

¼ teaspoon Celtic or pink Himalayan salt

¼ teaspoon freshly ground black pepper

1 clove garlic, minced

1 egg, beaten

Chopped fresh basil, for garnish

Preheat the oven to 425°F. Coat a baking sheet with coconut oil spray or line with foil.

Coat a medium pan with coconut oil spray and cook the sausage over medium-high heat, breaking it up with a wooden spoon, until no longer pink, about 5 minutes.

Meanwhile, with a spoon or melon baller, scoop out the flesh of each eggplant, leaving a ¼-inch-thick shell. Coarsely chop the flesh and add to the skillet with 2 teaspoons of the oil, the tomato, olives, onion, salt, and pepper. Cook, stirring occasionally, until the tomato and eggplant are softened and any liquid has evaporated, about 8 minutes. Add the garlic and cook for 1 minute more. Remove from the heat and let cool for 5 minutes. Mix in the egg.

Rub the remaining 2 teaspoons oil all over the eggplant shells. Divide the filling evenly among the shells and press in firmly. Place on the baking sheet and bake until the filling is hot and the eggplants are tender, about 25 minutes.

Serve sprinkled with basil.

TIP: *These boats can be grilled, too! If using Japanese eggplants: Coat a square of foil with coconut oil spray, place the foil on the grill grates over indirect heat, and set the stuffed eggplants on the foil. Grill, covered, until the filling is hot and the eggplants are tender, about 25 minutes. If using regular eggplants: Skip the foil and grill directly on the grates over indirect heat.*

# BLT STACKS

These little stacks serve up all the goodness of a BLT sandwich without the carbs. They're also as cute as they are tasty!

PREP TIME: 5 minutes
COOK TIME: 10 minutes
YIELD: 4 servings
PORTIONS: 1 protein, ½ fat, 1 vegetable

2 tablespoons Homemade Mayonnaise (page 76)

1 tablespoon chopped red onion

1 tablespoon chopped basil leaves

2 teaspoons fresh lemon juice

1 teaspoon Dijon mustard

1 teaspoon capers, chopped

4 slices uncured bacon

1 head butter lettuce, leaves separated

1 large heirloom tomato, cut into 4 slices

In a small bowl, stir together the mayonnaise, onion, basil, lemon juice, mustard, and capers. Set the aioli aside.

In a large skillet, cook the bacon over medium heat until crispy, 5 to 8 minutes. Drain on paper towels.

To assemble, stack the ingredients in this order: 1 butter lettuce leaf, 1 slice tomato, 1 slice bacon (cut in half). Repeat to make 3 more stacks.

Serve drizzled with the lemon-Dijon aioli.

**TIP:** *Alternatively, you can chop the tomato and layer the ingredients in an airtight container, keeping the aioli separate until ready to eat.*

# THAI-SPICED LAMB CHOPS

These curry-infused "lollipop" chops are lifesavers when you need to get dinner on the table quickly. Leftovers (if you have any!) make handy lunch box treats.

PREP TIME: 5 minutes

COOK TIME: 20 minutes

YIELD: 4 servings

PORTIONS: 1 protein, 1 fat

¼ cup coconut oil, melted

2 tablespoons fresh lime juice

1 tablespoon Thai green curry paste

2 cloves garlic, minced

1¾ pounds lamb rib chops (about 12)

Celtic or pink Himalayan salt

1 scallion, thinly sliced

Position a rack 4 inches below the broiler and preheat the broiler to high.

In a wide, shallow dish, combine the coconut oil, lime juice, curry paste, and garlic. Place the lamb chops in the mixture and marinate for 10 minutes, turning once.

Remove the chops from the marinade and arrange on a broiler pan. Sprinkle salt evenly on both sides. Broil, turning halfway through cooking, until the chops are nicely browned on both sides and a thermometer inserted in the center registers 145°F for medium-rare, about 8 minutes total.

Serve sprinkled with scallions.

## MAKE IT A 20

*Serve with Kamut: Cook 1 cup raw Kamut according to package directions in Asian Chicken Bone Broth (page 72) instead of water. Mix with chopped cilantro before serving.*

# *Fish*

Is there anything more beautiful than a melt-in-your-mouth salmon fillet straight off the grill, or a lobster tail dripping with clarified butter? Not in my book! And better yet, seafood is brimming with omega-3 fatty acids that make your skin cells vibrant and "bouncy."

When you can, choose fatty fish, which are the richest in omega-3s. If you're concerned about the mercury in fish—especially if you're pregnant or nursing—choose salmon, which is low in mercury, and avoid albacore tuna, mackerel, swordfish, shark, and tilefish.

To make sure you're buying high-quality seafood, look for fish with clear eyes and firm, shiny skin that bounces back when you touch it. Fresh fish smells like the ocean, but it doesn't smell *too* fishy. And fillets should be firm when you touch them—not falling apart. Wild-caught fish is best, but if that's not in your budget, farmed fish is just fine.

Once you buy your beautiful fish, get creative with it! With recipes ranging from Pesto Arctic Char and Vegetables en Papillote to Mussels with Tomato and Fennel Broth, now's your chance to become a gourmet seafood chef. And don't worry . . . you'll also find some basics, like grilled salmon, a crab cake salad, and even a fun twist on fish and chips.

# PESTO ARCTIC CHAR and VEGETABLES EN PAPILLOTE

It's fun to surprise dinner guests with these flavorful fillets, baked with pesto and veggies in parchment paper packages that you snip open at the table. If you can't find Arctic char, you can substitute salmon.

PREP TIME: 15 minutes
COOK TIME: 30 minutes

YIELD: 4 servings

PORTIONS: 1 protein, 1 fat, 1 vegetable

4 arctic char fillets (about 4 ounces each)

Celtic or pink Himalayan salt and freshly ground black pepper

¼ cup Pesto (page 82)

12 asparagus spears, woody ends trimmed, cut into 1-inch pieces

2 medium carrots, thinly sliced

1 large red bell pepper, thinly sliced

1 small yellow squash, halved lengthwise and thinly sliced crosswise into half-moons

1 small zucchini, halved lengthwise and thinly sliced crosswise into half-moons

2 tablespoons olive oil

Small basil leaves, for garnish

Position the racks in the upper and lower thirds of the oven and preheat to 375°F.

Lightly season the fillets on both sides with salt and pepper. Spread the pesto over the top of each fillet and set aside.

Cut 4 pieces of parchment paper, each measuring about 18 × 12 inches, and lay them on a clean work surface. Fold each in half crosswise, then open and lay flat, like a book.

In a medium bowl, toss the asparagus, carrots, bell pepper, yellow squash, and zucchini with the oil and sprinkle with salt and pepper. Divide the vegetables evenly among the pieces of parchment on one side of the fold. Lay a fillet on top of the vegetables and fold over the parchment. Fold over the open edges of parchment several times to form a seal that won't allow the steam to escape.

Transfer the packets to 2 large rimmed baking sheets and cook until the parchment puffs up, 10 to 12 minutes. (You may check the doneness of the fish by unfolding one edge and inserting a thin knife into the flesh for a couple seconds and then carefully touching the knife to your inner wrist or lip. The knife should feel warm, just above body temperature. If not, fold the parchment again and cook for 2 minutes more.)

Immediately place each packet on a plate and use kitchen shears to cut open the packets at the table. Sprinkle with fresh basil leaves.

# BAKED COCONUT SHRIMP with SPICY COCKTAIL SAUCE

These crispy, golden gems are perfect for dipping in a kicked-up version of my cocktail sauce. Total indulgence!

PREP TIME: 5 minutes
COOK TIME: 15 minutes

YIELD: 4 servings

PORTIONS: 1 protein, 2 fat

¾ cup unsweetened shredded coconut

¼ cup ground golden flaxseed

½ teaspoon Celtic or pink Himalayan salt

¼ cup ghee or coconut oil, melted and briefly cooled

1 pound large shrimp, peeled and deveined (tails left on)

½ recipe Cocktail Sauce (page 79)

1–2 teaspoons crab boil seasoning

Lemon wedges, for serving

Preheat the oven to 400°F. Set a wire rack inside a rimmed baking sheet and coat with coconut oil spray or brush with melted coconut oil.

In a medium bowl, combine the coconut, ground flax, and salt. Place the ghee in a separate bowl. Add the shrimp to the ghee, tossing to evenly coat. Working in batches, transfer the shrimp to the coconut mixture, turning to coat and pressing to adhere, if necessary. Place the shrimp on the wire rack. Bake until the coating is golden and the shrimp are cooked through (curled and opaque), about 10 minutes.

Meanwhile, in a small bowl, combine the cocktail sauce with 1 teaspoon of the crab boil seasoning. Taste and add more seasoning, if desired.

Serve the shrimp with the cocktail sauce and lemon wedges.

## MAKE IT A 20

*Serve with brown basmati rice: Cook 1 cup raw rice according to package directions, replacing half the water with unsweetened coconut milk.*

# GRILLED LOBSTER TAILS with GARLIC and HERB GHEE

Give halved lobster tails a quick cook on a hot grill, bathing them in garlicky ghee seasoned with fresh chives, tarragon, and lemon—fast, easy, and delicious.

PREP TIME: 10 minutes
COOK TIME: 15 minutes
YIELD: 4 servings
PORTIONS: 1 protein, 1 fat

- 4 tablespoons ghee, softened
- 1 tablespoon thinly sliced fresh chives
- 1 tablespoon finely chopped fresh tarragon
- 1 teaspoon finely grated lemon peel
- 1 clove garlic, minced
- Celtic or pink Himalayan salt and freshly ground black pepper
- 4 lobster tails (6–7 ounces each), thawed if frozen
- Lemon wedges, for serving

Preheat a gas or charcoal grill to medium-high heat.

In a small bowl, combine the ghee, chives, tarragon, lemon peel, garlic, and a pinch of salt and pepper. Using a fork, lightly mash all the ingredients together to release their flavors. Set aside.

Using kitchen shears, cut along the center of the back of the lobster tails from the opening to the tail fin. Turn the tail over and repeat the same cut on the bottom. Use a knife to cut through the meat to create two halves. Clean out the intestinal tract, if present.

Place the tails, shell side up, on the grill and close the lid. Grill until the meat of the tails is lightly marked, about 3 minutes. Turn the tails over. Dollop the ghee over the lobster meat, close the lid, and grill until the lobster meat is firm, moist, and opaque, 2 to 3 minutes more.

Serve with lemon wedges. The lobster can be served warm, at room temperature, or chilled as part of a lobster salad.

# WHOLE ROASTED BRANZINO with CAPER SAUCE

Branzino also goes by the name of European sea bass. Here, a simple sauce of capers, lemon juice, parsley, and pepper accents the delicate flavor of the fish.

PREP TIME: 10 minutes
COOK TIME: 20 minutes
YIELD: 4 servings
PORTIONS: 1 protein, 1 fat, 1 vegetable

1 whole branzino (4–6 pounds), cleaned and scaled with head and tail on (see Tip)

2 tablespoons olive oil

1 teaspoon Celtic or pink Himalayan salt

1 lemon, sliced

1 pint cherry tomatoes, halved

¼ pound thin green beans, halved

1 shallot, sliced

2 tablespoons ghee

2 tablespoons capers, rinsed and drained

2 tablespoons chopped fresh flat-leaf parsley

1 tablespoon fresh lemon juice

¼ teaspoon freshly ground black pepper

Preheat the oven to 425°F.

With a sharp knife, score the skin on both sides of the fish by making 3 or 4 shallow diagonal cuts. Rub 1 teaspoon of the oil on both sides of the fish. Sprinkle the fish on all sides and in the cavity with ½ teaspoon of the salt. Line the cavity with the lemon slices.

On a large baking sheet, combine the tomatoes, green beans, shallot, remaining ½ teaspoon salt, and remaining 1 tablespoon plus 2 teaspoons oil. Set the fish on the bed of vegetables. Bake until the fish is opaque, about 15 minutes.

Meanwhile, in a small saucepan, melt the ghee. Stir in the capers, parsley, lemon juice, and pepper and cook for 1 minute to heat through.

Serve the branzino and vegetables drizzled with the caper sauce.

TIP: *If you can't find a large branzino, look for two fish about 2 pounds each. Decrease the baking time to 10 to 12 minutes.*

# SEARED TUNA STEAKS with JICAMA SALSA

Citrusy jicama salsa is the perfect complement to barely-seared yellowfin tuna. If you're new to jicama, which stars in this salsa, you'll fall in love with its crunchy, slightly sweet taste.

PREP TIME: 15 minutes
COOK TIME: 1 hour 5 minutes

YIELD: 4 servings

PORTIONS: 1 protein, 1 fat, 1 fruit, 1 starchy vegetable

2 oranges

1 lime

½ pound jicama, peeled and grated (2 cups)

¼ red onion, finely chopped

¼ cup coarsely chopped fresh cilantro

½–1 fresh red chile or jalapeño pepper (see Tip), seeded and finely chopped (wear gloves when handling)

Celtic or pink Himalayan salt

4 albacore or yellowfin tuna steaks (6 ounces each, about 1-inch thick)

½ teaspoon freshly ground black pepper

1 tablespoon olive oil

Grate the peel from one of the oranges and the lime into a medium bowl.

To the bowl, add the jicama, onion, cilantro, chile pepper, and a pinch of salt. Over a separate bowl, segment the oranges (see Tip), then squeeze the membranes over the bowl of jicama to add all the juice. Slice the orange segments in half, then add them to the jicama with any collected juices. Gently toss, cover, and refrigerate for 1 hour.

Take the tuna out of the refrigerator 10 minutes before you're ready to cook it and season both sides with ½ teaspoon salt and the pepper.

In a large skillet, heat the oil over high heat. Add the tuna, sear for 2 minutes, and turn (the tuna should release easily). Sear the other side until desired doneness, 1 to 2 minutes more.

Serve each steak with ½ cup salsa.

TIP: *If you enjoy more heat, keep the seeds in the chile pepper.*

TO SEGMENT AN ORANGE: *Slice off the top and bottom so the orange can stand steadily. Use a sharp paring knife to cut the peel and white pith off the flesh, starting at the top and following down along the natural curve of the fruit inside the peel. Once it's peeled, hold the fruit in one hand over a bowl, then use the paring knife to cut between the flesh and the white membranes separating the individual segments, allowing these to fall into the bowl along with any juice.*

# FISH and CHIPS

This crusty, pan-fried fish is breaded with chopped almonds. Serve it with yummy root-vegetable chips.

PREP TIME: 15 minutes

COOK TIME: 30 minutes

YIELD: 4 servings

PORTIONS: 1 protein, 1 fat, 1 starchy vegetable

**For the chips:**

1 pound mixed root vegetables (yucca, sweet potatoes or yams, beets, celery root, rutabaga, turnip, carrots, parsnips), peeled and cut into wedges

Coconut oil spray

½ teaspoon Celtic or pink Himalayan salt

1 tablespoon apple cider vinegar, plus more for serving

**For the fish:**

2 egg whites, lightly beaten

1 cup finely chopped almonds

1 pound white fish (cod, turbot, haddock), about 1-inch thick, cut into 2- to 3-inch pieces

Coconut oil spray

*For the chips:* Preheat the oven to 400°F. Spray a large baking sheet with coconut oil spray and add the root vegetables. Sprinkle with the salt and bake, stirring once, until golden, about 30 minutes. Remove from the oven and toss with the vinegar.

*For the fish:* Spray a baking sheet with coconut oil spray. Set the eggs and almonds in their own shallow dishes. Dip the fish in the egg whites, allowing the excess to drip off, then coat the pieces in the almonds, turning the fish and pressing gently to adhere to all sides. Set on the prepared baking sheet.

Bake until the crust is golden and the fish is cooked through, about 10 to 15 minutes, rotating the baking sheets between the upper and lower oven racks halfway through baking.

Serve the fish with the roasted veggie chips and more cider vinegar, if desired.

# MUSSELS with TOMATO and FENNEL BROTH

This dish combines flavors of the sea with fresh tomatoes and a hint of fennel. Garnish it with fennel fronds for a lovely presentation.

PREP TIME: 10 minutes
COOK TIME: 20 minutes

YIELD: 4 servings

PORTIONS: 1 protein, ½ fat, 1 vegetable

1 tablespoon ghee

1 tablespoon olive oil

1 bulb fennel, trimmed, cored, and sliced (fronds reserved for garnish)

1 cup grape, pear, or cherry tomatoes, halved

2 cloves garlic, minced

1 cup Fish Bone Broth (page 69)

2 pounds mussels, rinsed and debearded (see Tip)

In a large skillet with a lid, heat the ghee and oil over medium heat until the ghee is melted. Add the fennel and cook until it starts to turn golden and softens, 8 to 10 minutes. Add the tomatoes and cook until broken down, 3 to 4 minutes. Add the garlic and stir until fragrant, 1 to 2 minutes more.

Stir in the broth and bring to a simmer. Add the mussels, scattering until they're nestled in the broth. Cover and steam until all the mussels open, about 5 minutes. (Discard any that do not.)

To serve, pour into a large bowl and garnish with fennel fronds, if desired.

TIP: *The beard is the mossy-looking bit that hangs off the mussel at the hinge, where the two shells join. It's not inedible, but it is a bit unpleasant. Not every mussel will have a beard, and all it takes is a little tug to pull it free. Tug toward the hinge of the mussel, and give it a wiggle to pull it free.*

### MAKE IT A 20

*Add a splash of white wine to the broth or serve with oven-baked fries and Homemade Mayonnaise (page 76).*

# GRILLED SALMON with SPICED BLUEBERRY SAUCE

Fresh blueberries, simmered with shallots, garlic, red wine vinegar, and spices, make a sweet and savory sauce for salmon steaks. Add lime wedges for a finishing touch.

PREP TIME: 10 minutes
COOK TIME: 20 minutes

YIELD: 4 servings

PORTIONS: 1 protein, 1 fat, ½ fruit

- 1 tablespoon olive oil
- 1 shallot, finely chopped
- 1 clove garlic, minced
- 1 cup blueberries (6 ounces)
- 1 tablespoon red wine vinegar
- ¼ teaspoon ground cardamom
- ¼ teaspoon ground coriander
- ¼ teaspoon ground ginger
- ½ teaspoon Celtic or pink Himalayan salt
- 4 salmon steaks (about 1½ pounds)
- ¼ teaspoon freshly ground black pepper
- 4 lime wedges, for serving

In a medium saucepan, heat the oil over medium heat. Add the shallot and cook, stirring, until it starts to soften, about 3 minutes. Add the garlic and cook for 1 minute more. Deglaze the pan with ¼ cup water and reduce the heat to medium-low. Add the blueberries, red wine vinegar, cardamom, coriander, ginger, and ¼ teaspoon of the salt. Simmer, crushing half the berries, until thickened, about 10 minutes. Remove from the heat and cover to keep warm.

Preheat a gas grill or grill pan to medium-high heat. Lightly oil the grill grates (or coat the grill pan with coconut oil spray). Season one side of each salmon steak with the remaining ¼ teaspoon salt and the pepper. Grill, seasoning side down, for 4 minutes. Turn and grill until just opaque, 3 to 4 minutes more.

Serve with 1 to 2 tablespoons sauce per steak and a lime wedge.

## MAKE IT A 20

*Serve with toasted herby millet: Toast ½ cup millet in a dry saucepan until fragrant (3 to 5 minutes), then cook according to package directions in Chicken Bone Broth (page 65) or Fish Bone Broth (page 69) instead of water. Stir in ½ cup chopped fresh herbs (parsley, cilantro, thyme, or chives) before serving.*

# 4-CITRUS SCALLOP CEVICHE

The scallops in this dish "cook" in a mixture of citrus juices, garlic, and chile. To finish the dish, simply toss with avocado, mango, and cilantro.

PREP TIME: 15 minutes

COOK TIME: 2 hours

YIELD: 4 servings

PORTIONS: 1 protein, 1 fat, 1 fruit

½ cup fresh grapefruit juice

½ cup fresh orange juice

¼ cup fresh lemon juice

¼ cup fresh lime juice

½ medium red onion, halved lengthwise, then thinly sliced

1 clove garlic, mashed to a paste with the side of a chef's knife

½ small habanero chile (optional, or use less for less heat), seeded and finely chopped (wear gloves when handling)

Celtic or pink Himalayan salt and freshly ground black pepper

1 pound bay scallops (see Tip), halved if large

1 avocado

1 mango

¼ cup finely chopped fresh cilantro

In a large glass, plastic, or stainless steel bowl, stir together the citrus juices, onion, garlic, chile (if using), and a pinch of salt and pepper. Add the scallops and toss well. Cover and refrigerate for at least 2 and up to 16 hours.

Just before serving, dice the avocado and mango and toss into the ceviche mixture along with the cilantro.

Using a slotted spoon, serve in chilled glasses or bowls, drizzling some of the liquid over the ceviche.

TIP: *Bay scallops are small, about the size of your thumbnail. If they're out of season or unavailable, use sea scallops cut into quarters.*

# CRAB CAKE SALAD

With not a breadcrumb in sight, the crab in this salad is low-carb, guilt-free, and oh so tasty. It's tucked into a salad of lightly dressed greens and tomato slices.

PREP TIME: 10 minutes
COOK TIME: 20 minutes
YIELD: 4 servings
PORTIONS: 1 protein, 1 fat, 1 vegetable

- 1 pound jumbo lump crabmeat, picked over
- 3 tablespoons Homemade Mayonnaise (page 76)
- 3 tablespoons finely chopped red onion
- 3 tablespoons finely chopped red bell pepper
- 2 tablespoons finely chopped fresh flat-leaf parsley
- ¼ cup plus 2 tablespoons fresh lemon juice
- Celtic or pink Himalayan salt and freshly ground black pepper
- 1 tablespoon extra-virgin olive oil, plus more for drizzling
- 4 cups baby arugula
- ¼ cup very loosely packed basil leaves, thinly sliced
- 1 large heirloom tomato, cut into 4 thick slices

In a medium bowl, combine the crab, mayonnaise, onion, bell pepper, parsley, and ¼ cup of the lemon juice. Toss gently, being careful not to break up the meat. Season to taste with salt and black pepper. Marinate for 10 to 15 minutes at room temperature. Put the crab in a fine-mesh sieve set over a medium bowl and drain for at least 5 minutes. (Discard the marinade.)

In another medium bowl, whisk together the oil, the remaining 2 tablespoons lemon juice, and a pinch of salt and pepper. Add the arugula and basil and toss to coat with the dressing.

To serve, divide the greens into mounds on 4 small plates. Top each with a tomato slice (see Tip). Season the tomatoes with salt and pepper and top each with one-quarter of the crab mixture. Drizzle with a little olive oil before serving.

TIP: *If you want to get fancy, set a 2½-inch round cookie cutter on top of the tomato slice. Pack the crab salad mixture into the cookie cutter and press lightly. Carefully remove the cookie cutter.*

# Vegetarian

Yes! You *can* do the Bone Broth Diet if you're a vegetarian (see page 39). And even if you're not a vegetarian, a nonmeat meal can be a fun change of pace.

Just remember that you do want to have protein at every meal—so unless you're making a vegetarian recipe that includes eggs, be sure to add some protein on the side. Nut butters and protein powders are good sources, and so are beans (which aren't allowed on the basic diet but are okay on the vegetarian version).

By the way, if you're hosting a dinner party for vegetarian guests, I recommend the Roasted Cauliflower Steaks with Yemeni Hot Sauce and the Naked Beet Sliders. *Très élégant!*

# NORI ROLLS

To make this vegetarian "sushi," roll up avocado, marinated shiitake mushrooms, scallions, and cucumber in nori sheets and slice like sushi rolls. Serve with a wasabi/rice vinegar dipping sauce.

PREP TIME: 15 minutes
COOK TIME: 15 minutes
YIELD: 4 servings
PORTIONS: 1 fat, 1 vegetable

¼ cup rice vinegar

1 tablespoon toasted sesame oil

2 cloves garlic, minced

2 teaspoons finely chopped fresh ginger

¼ pound shiitake mushroom caps, sliced

8 sheets nori

½ avocado, pitted, peeled, and sliced lengthwise

4 scallions, thinly sliced

1 English cucumber, peeled and cut into ¼-inch-thick, 2-inch-long strips

¼ teaspoon wasabi powder or grated fresh horseradish

In a medium bowl, stir together the rice vinegar, sesame oil, garlic, and ginger. Set aside half of the mixture for the dipping sauce. Add the mushrooms to the remaining vinegar mixture and stir to coat.

In a medium skillet, cook the mushrooms over medium heat until they soften and release some liquid, 3 to 5 minutes. Set aside to cool.

To assemble, place 1 nori sheet on a dry surface. Spoon a few mushrooms on the bottom of the sheet, then top with slices of avocado, scallion, and cucumber. Roll up tightly and lightly wet the edge with water to seal the roll. Slice crosswise into 6 pieces. Repeat with the remaining ingredients.

Stir the wasabi powder into the reserved sauce and serve with the nori rolls.

## MAKE IT A 20

*Add sushi rice cooked in Asian Chicken Bone Broth (page 72).*

# NAKED BEET SLIDERS

Shredded beets and zucchini stand in for the beef in these bite-size treats. Serve atop a slice of tomato slathered with creamy homemade Dijonnaise.

PREP TIME: 15 minutes

COOK TIME: 20 minutes

YIELD: 2 servings

PORTIONS: 1 fat, 1 vegetable

2 medium beets, peeled

1 small zucchini

1 tablespoon ground flaxseed

½ teaspoon smoked paprika

½ teaspoon dried oregano

Celtic or pink Himalayan salt and freshly ground black pepper

¼ cup Homemade Mayonnaise (page 76)

1 tablespoon Dijon mustard

2 small tomatoes, sliced

Preheat the oven to 350°F. Coat a baking sheet with coconut oil spray.

Shred the beets on the large holes of a box grater (you should have about 2 cups). Grate the zucchini in the same way.

In a medium bowl, combine the beets, zucchini, ground flaxseed, paprika, oregano, and salt and pepper to taste. Form into 8 patties about 2½ inches wide. Place the patties on the prepared baking sheet and bake until golden and crisp, turning once during cooking, about 20 minutes.

Meanwhile, in a small bowl, combine the mayonnaise and mustard.

To serve, top tomato slices with the beet sliders and a dollop of Dijonnaise.

# PESTO EGGPLANT ROLL-UPS with ROASTED RED PEPPERS

In this fun recipe, pesto, red pepper, and spinach snuggle up together inside eggplant "wraps." This dish is a big hit at dinner parties, and you can make it ahead of time and add the dressing just before serving.

PREP TIME: 5 minutes

COOK TIME: 15 minutes

YIELD: 4 servings

PORTIONS: 1 fat, 1 vegetable

- 1 large eggplant (1¼–1½ pounds), cut lengthwise into 8 slabs, about ¼-inch thick
- 4 tablespoons Pesto (page 82)
- 1 cup baby spinach
- ½ cup jarred roasted red pepper strips, drained and patted dry
- 2 tablespoons olive oil
- 1 tablespoon fresh lemon juice
- 1 tablespoon chopped fresh basil
- ¼ teaspoon Celtic or pink Himalayan salt

Preheat a gas grill or grill pan to medium-high heat. Brush the grates with oil or coat the grill pan with coconut oil spray.

Lightly coat both sides of the eggplant slices with coconut oil spray. Grill the eggplant until well marked and tender, 4 to 5 minutes per side. Transfer to a work surface to cool slightly.

Brush one side of each eggplant slice with ½ tablespoon pesto. Divide the spinach and roasted pepper among the eggplant slices, placing them on the bottom third. Roll up each slice from the bottom and place, seam side down, on a platter.

In a small bowl, whisk together the olive oil, lemon juice, basil, and salt. Drizzle over the rolls and serve immediately. (Alternatively, cover the rolls without the dressing, refrigerate, and bring back to room temperature before serving with the dressing.)

**Variation:**

Lightly coat an 8 × 8-inch baking dish with coconut oil spray. Nestle the rolls in the dish, seam side down. Cover with foil and bake at 350°F until hot, about 15 minutes.

## MAKE IT A 20

*Top with the dressing and serve with a side of cooked ancient-grain pasta or brown rice pasta mixed with a bit of additional pesto.*

# ROASTED CAULIFLOWER STEAKS with YEMENI HOT SAUCE

Pan-roasted spices turn tender slices of roasted cauliflower into a savory entree. Add extra zing with my fiery Middle Eastern hot-pepper sauce.

PREP TIME: 10 minutes

COOK TIME: 35 minutes

YIELD: 4 servings

PORTIONS: 1 fat, 1 vegetable

- 1 teaspoon cumin seeds
- ½ teaspoon coriander seeds
- ½ teaspoon Celtic or pink Himalayan salt
- ¼ teaspoon black peppercorns
- 1 large head cauliflower, bottom trimmed and outer leaves removed
- ¼ cup olive oil, plus more for brushing
- 3 cloves garlic, coarsely chopped
- 1 or 2 serrano peppers, seeded (if desired) and coarsely chopped (wear gloves when handling)
- 1 cup parsley leaves
- 1 cup cilantro leaves

Preheat the oven to 400°F. Line a baking sheet with parchment paper or foil.

In a small skillet, combine the cumin seeds, coriander seeds, salt, and peppercorns and toast over medium heat until fragrant, about 2 minutes. Cool, transfer to a food processor or spice grinder, and crush to a fine powder. Measure out 1 teaspoon and set aside. (Leave the rest of the mixture in the food processor.)

Set the cauliflower stem side down on a work surface and cut vertically into 1-inch-thick slabs. Arrange in a single layer on the baking sheet and brush the tops with some oil. Sprinkle the reserved 1 teaspoon spice mixture over the cauliflower and bake until tender and golden, 35 to 40 minutes.

Meanwhile, to the food processor with the remaining spices, add the garlic and serrano pepper and process until a paste forms. Add the parsley and cilantro and process until coarsely chopped. With the machine running, slowly pour in the ¼ cup oil and ¼ cup water to form a loose mixture. Taste and season with more salt if necessary.

Serve the sauce over the hot cauliflower steaks.

## CHAPTER 8

# Superhero Sidekicks:

## *Yummy Salads and Sides to Brighten Your Plate*

As a kid, you probably hated hearing "Eat your vegetables." That's because frequently, these vegetables were just *awful*—especially the lumpy, soggy ones on your school lunch trays. Since then, there's a good chance you've eaten more than your share of frozen vegetables packaged in plastic bags, covered in preservative-laden sauces, and zapped in the microwave.

As a result, you may be pretty reluctant when I tell you to load up your plate with greens. But trust me: Once you start preparing vegetables in ways that make their flavors sing, you're going to become a fan. And when you realize how much fat-burning, wrinkle-erasing power those colorful veggies contain, you'll *really* grow to appreciate them.

But what if you're already into veggies? In that case, I have *more* ways for you to fall in love with these fantastic foods. I'm going to share adventurous new ways to use them—for instance, in my Fennel-Grapefruit Salad with Olives and my Parsnip, Rutabaga, and Sweet Potato Puree. You'll also discover fun new twists on fruit, like my tostones.

So read on . . . and let me introduce you to a cornucopia of delicious recipes that will turn your side dishes into full-fledged stars.

### A QUICK REMINDER ABOUT "ENERGY VEGGIES"

In Chapter 3, I distinguished between starchy and nonstarchy vegetables. That's because you'll want to use them in different ways.

Nonstarchy vegetables are very low in carbs, so you can eat them like crazy. In fact, I want you to fill your plate with as many as you can eat. You simply can't overdo it.

Starchy vegetables, on the other hand, do pack some carbs. They're far, far better for you than other carbs like sugar and grains, but they'll still raise your blood sugar. So I want you to limit these veggies, eating them only when you need a boost of energy—for instance, on days when you've exercised strenuously. Think of them as very occasional "power-ups."

## A NOTE ABOUT GUT-HEALING VEGGIES

You already know that veggies are packed with vitamins, minerals, and phytonutrients. But did you know that they also help you grow a beautiful "gut garden?" They do this in two ways:

- **They populate your gut with good bugs.** Fermented vegetables like kimchi, pickles, and sauerkraut are *probiotics* packed with live, beneficial microbes. These little heroes will settle happily into your ecosystem, helping to build a diverse and well-balanced microbiome.

- **They build fertile soil for good bugs.** To grow a fabulous outdoor garden, you need great soil. And guess what: It's the same story in your gut! Trillions and trillions of good microbes live in your GI tract, and they need rich, healthy soil in order to flourish. That's where *prebiotics* come in, because they're high in the soluble fiber your gut microbes love to eat. Great prebiotic vegetables include onions, garlic, asparagus, leeks, Jerusalem artichokes, and jicama (check out my Kohlrabi, Jicama, and Carrot Slaw!).

So load up on probiotic and prebiotic foods, as well as all the other beautiful, nutrient-packed vegetables and fruits you can savor on my diet. If you're a "veggie skeptic," you're going to fall in love with them . . . and if you're a long-time veggie fan, you're going to fall in love all over again!

# GRILLED GARDEN SALAD with GREEN GODDESS DRESSING

Romaine lettuce grills beautifully because it's so robust. In this recipe, you'll toss lightly charred lettuce with tomatoes, cucumbers, and chives, and top it all off with my Green Goddess dressing and a sprinkle of walnuts.

PREP TIME: 5 minutes

COOK TIME: 10 minutes

YIELD: 4 servings

PORTIONS: 1 fat, 2 vegetable

- 2 heads romaine lettuce, halved lengthwise, root end intact
- 2 teaspoons olive oil
- ¼ teaspoon Celtic or pink Himalayan salt
- ¼ teaspoon freshly ground black pepper
- 1 large tomato, chopped, or 1 cup cherry tomatoes, halved
- ½ English cucumber, chopped
- 2 tablespoons chopped fresh chives
- ½ cup Green Goddess Dressing (from California Plate, page 117)
- ½ cup coarsely chopped walnuts

Preheat a gas or charcoal grill to medium-high heat. Brush the lettuce with the oil. Sprinkle with salt and pepper. Place the lettuce on the grill grates and grill until lightly charred and wilted on all sides, 2 to 4 minutes. Remove from the grill and coarsely chop, discarding the root end. Transfer to a serving bowl and gently toss with the tomato, cucumber, and chives.

To serve, divide among 4 plates, drizzle with the dressing, and sprinkle with walnuts.

# FENNEL-GRAPEFRUIT SALAD
## with OLIVES

To make this quick salad, toss segmented ruby reds with thinly sliced fennel, chopped olives, and chopped mint. Then whisk the juice of the grapefruit with oil and rice vinegar and drizzle on top.

PREP TIME: 10 minutes
COOK TIME: 10 minutes
YIELD: 4 servings
PORTIONS: ½ fat, 1 fruit

- 2 ruby red grapefruit
- 1 large bulb fennel, trimmed, cored, and thinly sliced
- ¼ cup kalamata or niçoise olives, pitted and chopped
- ¼ cup chopped fresh mint
- 1 tablespoon chopped fresh tarragon
- 2 tablespoons avocado or olive oil
- 1 tablespoon rice vinegar
- ¼ teaspoon freshly ground black pepper

Segment the grapefruit over a small bowl (see Tip). Squeeze the juice from the membranes into the bowl. Transfer the segments to a medium bowl and gently toss with the fennel, olives, mint, and tarragon. Whisk the oil, vinegar, and pepper into the juice. Drizzle over the fennel mixture, tossing gently to coat well.

TIP: *To segment a grapefruit, slice off the top and bottom so it can stand steadily. Use a sharp paring knife to cut the peel and white pith off the flesh, starting at the top and following down along the natural curve of the fruit inside the peel. Once peeled, hold the fruit in one hand over a bowl, then use the paring knife to cut between the flesh and the white membranes separating the individual segments, allowing these to fall into the bowl along with any juice.*

# GREEK CUCUMBER, TOMATO, and RED ONION SALAD with RED WINE–OREGANO VINAIGRETTE

This rustic no-greens salad complements any entree. Save the leftovers because it's even better the next day.

PREP TIME: 10 minutes
COOK TIME: 5 minutes
YIELD: 4 servings
PORTIONS: ½ fat, 1 vegetable

¼ cup red wine vinegar

2 tablespoons extra-virgin olive oil

1 teaspoon dried oregano

Celtic or pink Himalayan salt and freshly ground black pepper

1½ pounds cucumbers (about 3 medium), peeled, halved lengthwise, seeded, and thickly sliced

1 pint cherry tomatoes, halved

½ red onion, thinly sliced

2 tablespoons chopped fresh dill

In a large bowl, whisk together the vinegar, oil, oregano, ½ teaspoon salt, and ¼ teaspoon pepper. Add the cucumbers, tomatoes, onion, and dill and toss to coat. Just before serving, adjust the seasoning to taste with more salt and pepper.

# KOHLRABI, JICAMA,
## and CARROT SLAW

Tired of the same-old, same-old cabbage slaw? Then surprise
your tastebuds with this sweet, crunchy variation.

PREP TIME: 10 minutes

COOK TIME: 1 hour

YIELD: 4 servings

PORTIONS: 1 fat, 1 starchy
vegetable

- 2 tablespoons red wine
  vinegar
- 1 teaspoon celery seeds
- ½ teaspoon Celtic or pink
  Himalayan salt
- ¼ teaspoon freshly ground
  black pepper
- 2 tablespoons avocado oil
- 1 medium kohlrabi, peeled
- 1 small jicama, peeled
- 2 medium carrots, peeled
- ¼ cup unsalted roasted
  pumpkin seeds

In a large bowl, whisk together the vinegar, celery seeds, salt,
and pepper. While whisking, drizzle in the avocado oil. On the
large holes of a box grater, shred the kohlrabi, jicama, and
carrots. Add to the bowl and toss to coat with the dressing. Let
sit for at least 1 hour to meld the flavors. Sprinkle with pumpkin
seeds just before serving.

# CAULIFLOWER "RICE" 3 WAYS

From fried rice to pilaf to risotto, cauliflower can do anything rice can do—and I think it tastes even better! Here are my riffs on three classic rice recipes.

## Fried Rice

PREP TIME: 5 minutes
COOK TIME: 15 minutes
YIELD: 4 servings
PORTIONS: ¼ protein, ¼ fat, 1 vegetable

1 medium head cauliflower, cut into florets (about 4 cups)

1 tablespoon toasted sesame oil

4 scallions, very thinly sliced (whites and greens kept separate)

1 large carrot, finely chopped

2 cloves garlic, minced

2 eggs, beaten

3 tablespoons coconut aminos

½ cup mung bean sprouts

In a food processor, pulse the cauliflower florets until they resemble small grains of rice.

In a large skillet, heat the sesame oil over medium heat. Add the scallion whites, carrot, and garlic and stir-fry until fragrant, about 5 minutes. Add the cauliflower and cook, stirring constantly, until the cauliflower is tender but not mushy, about 5 minutes.

Push the cauliflower mixture to the sides, leaving the center clear. Add the eggs and scramble until fully cooked, about 2 minutes. Stir everything together, then stir in the coconut aminos, scallion greens, and sprouts. Serve immediately.

# Rice Pilaf with Carrots and Pine Nuts

PREP TIME: 10 minutes

COOK TIME: 20 minutes

YIELD: 4 servings

PORTIONS: 1 fat, 1 vegetable

- 1 medium head cauliflower, cut into florets (about 4 cups)
- 2 tablespoons coconut or olive oil
- 1 yellow onion, finely chopped
- 2 carrots, finely chopped
- ½ teaspoon cumin seeds
- ½ teaspoon freshly ground black pepper
- ¼ teaspoon Celtic or pink Himalayan salt
- ¼ cup toasted pine nuts
- ¼ cup chopped fresh flat-leaf parsley
- 1 tablespoon chopped fresh mint
- 2 teaspoons grated orange peel
- 1 tablespoon fresh orange juice

In a food processor, pulse the cauliflower florets until they resemble small grains of rice.

In a large skillet, heat the oil over medium heat. Add the onion and carrots and cook, stirring, until beginning to brown and soften, about 8 minutes. Add the cumin seeds, pepper, and salt and toast for 1 minute. Add ½ cup water and stir to distribute. Add the cauliflower and cook, stirring, until tender, about 5 minutes.

To serve, sprinkle with the pine nuts, parsley, mint, orange peel, and orange juice.

# Cauliflower "Rice" Risotto with Wild Mushrooms

PREP TIME: 10 minutes
COOK TIME: 20 minutes
YIELD: 4 servings
PORTION: 1 vegetable

1 medium head cauliflower, cut into florets (about 4 cups)

1 tablespoon ghee or olive oil

1 small onion, finely chopped

4 ounces mixed wild mushrooms, chopped

¼ cup Chicken Bone Broth (page 65) or water

2 tablespoons nutritional yeast (see Tips)

½ teaspoon Celtic or pink Himalayan salt

¼ teaspoon freshly ground black pepper

In a food processor, pulse the cauliflower florets until they resemble small grains of rice.

In a medium saucepan, warm the ghee over medium heat. Add the onion and cook until softened, about 5 minutes. Add the mushrooms and cook until they release their liquid, about 5 minutes. Stir in the cauliflower and broth. Cover and cook until the cauliflower is tender, about 10 minutes. Stir in the nutritional yeast, salt, and pepper and serve.

**TIPS:**

*Nutritional yeast flakes can be found in the natural foods section of most supermarkets. Do not confuse them with brewer's yeast, which is sometimes labeled as nutritional yeast.*

*Raw cauliflower "rice" can be made ahead and frozen. After processing or grating, simply transfer to freezer storage bags or containers. If pan-frying or roasting, thaw it first on the countertop; if steaming, use it straight from the freezer.*

# PARSNIP, RUTABAGA, and SWEET POTATO PUREE

Bone broth and a splash of coconut make this mash rich and creamy, while herbs add brightness. You can make this ahead and reheat it just before serving.

PREP TIME: 10 minutes
COOK TIME: 20 minutes
YIELD: 4 servings
PORTIONS: ¼ fat, 1 starchy vegetable

- 2 parsnips, peeled and sliced
- 1 medium rutabaga (yellow turnip), peeled and cut into ½-inch pieces
- 1 medium sweet potato, peeled and cut into ½-inch pieces
- ¼ cup Chicken Bone Broth (page 65)
- 2 tablespoons coconut milk or ghee
- ½ teaspoon Celtic or pink Himalayan salt
- 2 teaspoons chopped fresh chives
- 2 teaspoons chopped fresh thyme or ½ teaspoon dried
- 1 teaspoon chopped fresh sage or ¼ teaspoon dried

Bring a large pot of lightly salted water to a boil. Add the parsnips, rutabaga, and sweet potato and boil until tender, 12 to 15 minutes. Drain and transfer to a food processor. (Alternatively, return to the pot and mash with a potato masher.) Add the broth, coconut milk, and salt. Process or mash until smooth. Pulse or stir in the chives, thyme, and sage. Serve warm.

# SRIRACHA-GLAZED TURNIPS

Turnips turn sweet and spicy when you pan-roast them in Sriracha-laced ghee. I like to double this recipe because it keeps well.

PREP TIME: 5 minutes
COOK TIME: 15 minutes

YIELD: 4 servings

PORTIONS: ¼ fat, 1 starchy vegetable

1 pound small turnips (such as Hakurei), trimmed and halved or quartered

1 tablespoon ghee

1 tablespoon Sriracha sauce (or more to taste)

½ teaspoon Celtic or pink Himalayan salt

In a large skillet with a lid, arrange the turnips in a single layer and add ½ cup water. Bring to a boil over high heat, cover, and cook until the turnips are tender, 8 to 10 minutes. Uncover and allow any extra water to evaporate. Stir in the ghee and Sriracha and cook until the ghee melts, about 1 minute more. Stir to coat the turnips in the sauce, season with salt, and serve.

# SIZZLING SESAME SCALLIONS

Scallions, which typically play a supporting role in recipes, take a star turn here. Sesame seeds and sesame oil give them a refreshing nutty flavor.

PREP TIME: 10 minutes

COOK TIME: 15 minutes

YIELD: 4 servings

PORTIONS: ½ fat, ¼ vegetable

- 2 tablespoons fresh lemon juice
- 1½ teaspoons toasted sesame oil
- 1 teaspoon gluten-free hot-pepper sauce or ¼ teaspoon crushed red-pepper flakes
- ¼ teaspoon Celtic or pink Himalayan salt
- ¼ cup sesame seeds
- 2 bunches scallions, cut crosswise into 1-inch lengths (halve any larger ones lengthwise first)

In a medium bowl, whisk together the lemon juice, 1 teaspoon of the sesame oil, hot-pepper sauce, and salt. Stir in the sesame seeds, then the scallions. Heat a large skillet over medium heat. Pour the mixture into the skillet and cook, stirring occasionally, until the scallions have browned and the sesame seeds have toasted, 7 to 8 minutes. Stir in the remaining ½ teaspoon sesame oil and serve.

## MAKE IT A 20

*Sweeten the pot by adding 1 teaspoon raw honey to the sauce.*

# TOSTONES with GARLIC and LIME

Tostones, which are hugely popular in South America, are twice-fried plantains. They're crunchy on the outside and tender on the inside, and the garlic and lime in this recipe add a punch of flavor.

PREP TIME: 5 minutes

COOK TIME: 15 minutes

YIELD: 4 servings

PORTIONS: 1 fat, 1 starchy vegetable

¼ cup olive oil

2 green plantains, peeled and cut into 1-inch-thick slices

2 cloves garlic, smashed

¼ teaspoon Celtic or pink Himalayan salt

Lime wedges, for serving

In a large skillet, heat 2 tablespoons of the oil over medium-high heat. Add the plantains and cook until they begin to brown, turning once, about 5 minutes. Remove from the heat and transfer to a cutting board.

Use the flat bottom of a mug, can of beans, or a small skillet to press and flatten the plantain slices.

Add the remaining 2 tablespoons oil and garlic to the skillet and heat over medium-high heat. Return the plantains to the skillet and cook, turning once, until they are crisped and brown, about 5 minutes. Sprinkle with salt and serve with lime wedges.

# ROASTED BROCCOLI with LEMON-CHILE SAUCE and ANCHOVY CRUMBLES

Humble broccoli gets a chance to shine in this quick-prep recipe. The anchovies add crunch and a rich, salty flavor.

PREP TIME: 5 minutes

COOK TIME: 20 minutes

YIELD: 4 servings

PORTIONS: 1 fat, 2 vegetable

- 2 large heads broccoli, cut into bite-size florets (see Tip)
- Coconut oil spray
- ½ teaspoon Celtic or pink Himalayan salt
- ½ jar (3.5 to 4.5 ounces) anchovies in olive oil
- 2 tablespoons coconut flour
- 3 tablespoons ghee
- 4 cloves garlic, minced
- ¼ cup Chicken Bone Broth (page 65)
- Juice of 1 lemon
- ¼–½ teaspoon crushed red-pepper flakes (to taste)

Preheat the oven to 425°F.

Arrange the broccoli florets on a baking sheet sprayed with coconut oil spray. Lightly spray the florets with more coconut oil spray and sprinkle with salt. Roast, undisturbed, until dark golden in most places, 20 to 25 minutes.

Meanwhile, in a small skillet, combine the anchovies with their oil and the flour. Cook over medium heat, breaking up the mixture with a wooden spoon, until small, crunchy brown crumbs form, 7 to 8 minutes. Transfer to a plate and wipe out the skillet.

Place the skillet over medium-low heat and melt the ghee. Add the garlic and cook until golden and very fragrant, about 1 minute. Add the broth, lemon juice, and pepper flakes and reduce to about ⅓ cup, 2 to 3 minutes.

Serve the broccoli drizzled with the sauce and topped with the anchovy crumbles.

TIP: *Don't toss the broccoli stems! They have just as many nutrients as the florets. Peel the tough outer layer and chop the creamy core. Roast with the florets.*

## MAKE IT A 20

*Add a splash of white wine to the sauce when you add the bone broth.*

# BRAISED BRUSSELS SPROUTS
## with BACON

Bacon makes everything fabulous—including these skillet-braised and broth-simmered sprouts. A thyme and mustard sauce adds a piquant note.

PREP TIME: 10 minutes

COOK TIME: 20 minutes

YIELD: 4 servings

PORTIONS: ½ protein, 1 vegetable

4 slices uncured bacon

1 pound medium Brussels sprouts, trimmed and halved

1 large shallot, thinly sliced

¼ teaspoon Celtic or pink Himalayan salt

¼ teaspoon freshly ground black pepper

⅓ cup Chicken Bone Broth (page 65)

2 teaspoons Dijon mustard

1½ teaspoons chopped fresh thyme

In a large skillet, cook the bacon over medium heat until crisp, about 8 minutes. Remove the bacon to a plate lined with paper towels. Crumble when cool.

Add the Brussels sprouts to the skillet, cut side down. Cook, undisturbed, until the sprouts start to take on color, about 2 minutes. Add the shallot, tossing to combine, and cook until the shallot begins to soften, about 2 minutes. Sprinkle with salt and pepper. Add ¼ cup of the broth to the skillet, cover, and cook until the Brussels sprouts are crisp-tender, about 3 minutes more.

In a small bowl, combine the mustard, thyme, and remaining broth. Stir the sauce into the Brussels sprouts. Cook, stirring, until well combined, about 1 minute.

Serve the sprouts topped with the crumbled bacon.

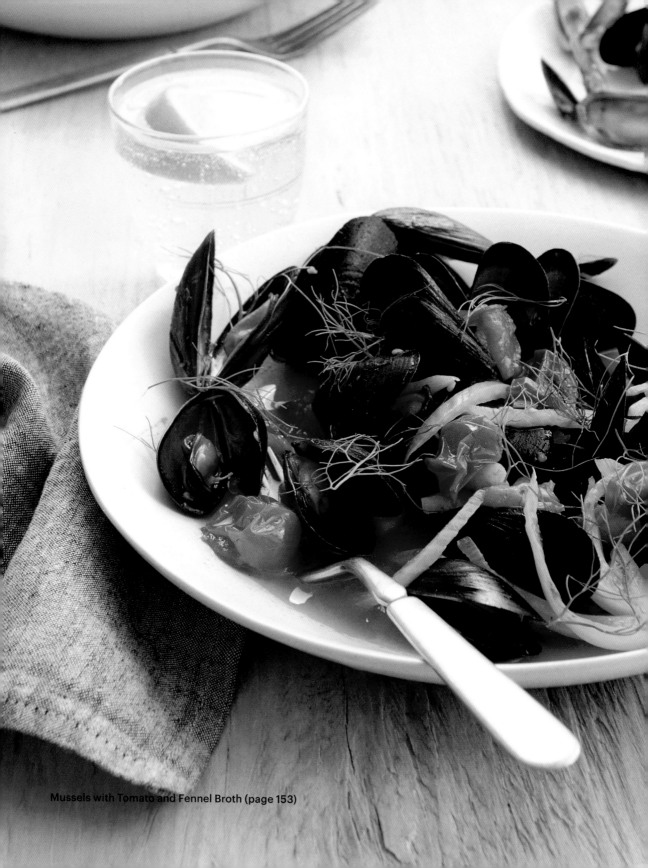

Mussels with Tomato and Fennel Broth (page 153)

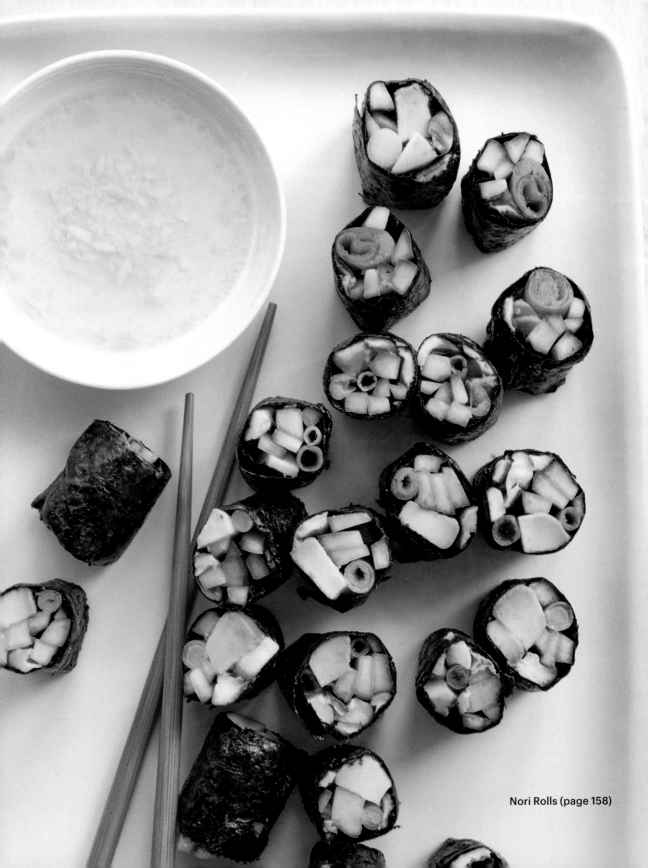

Nori Rolls (page 158)

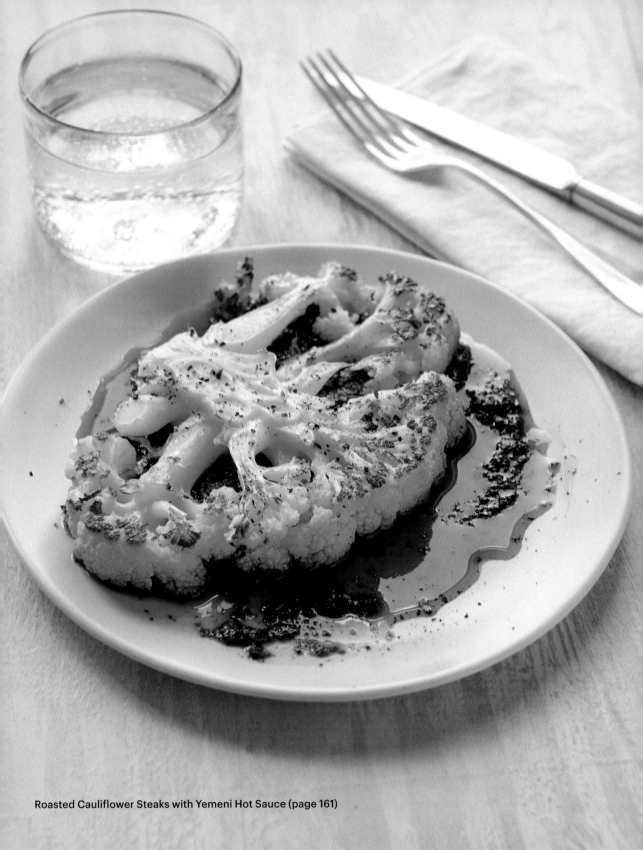

Roasted Cauliflower Steaks with Yemeni Hot Sauce (page 161)

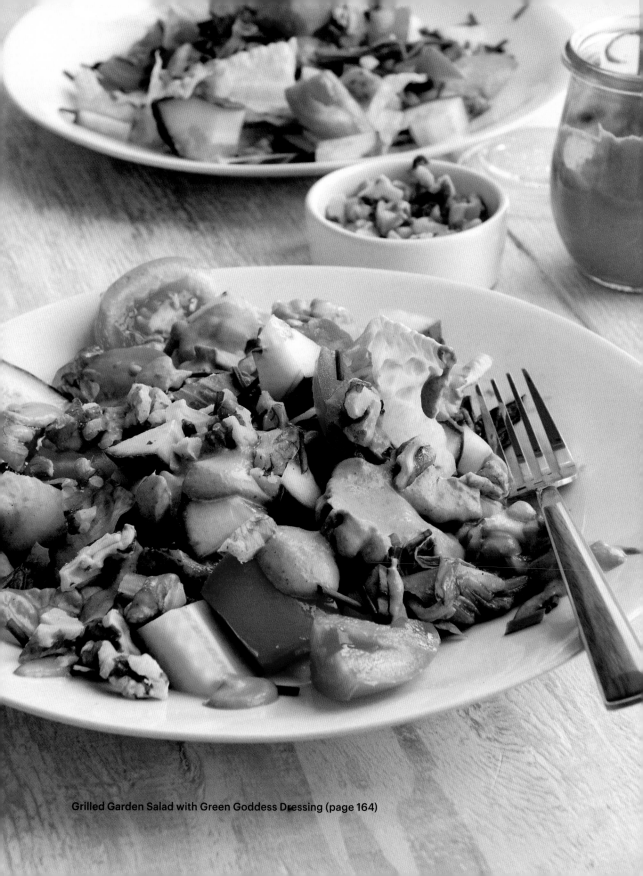

Grilled Garden Salad with Green Goddess Dressing (page 164)

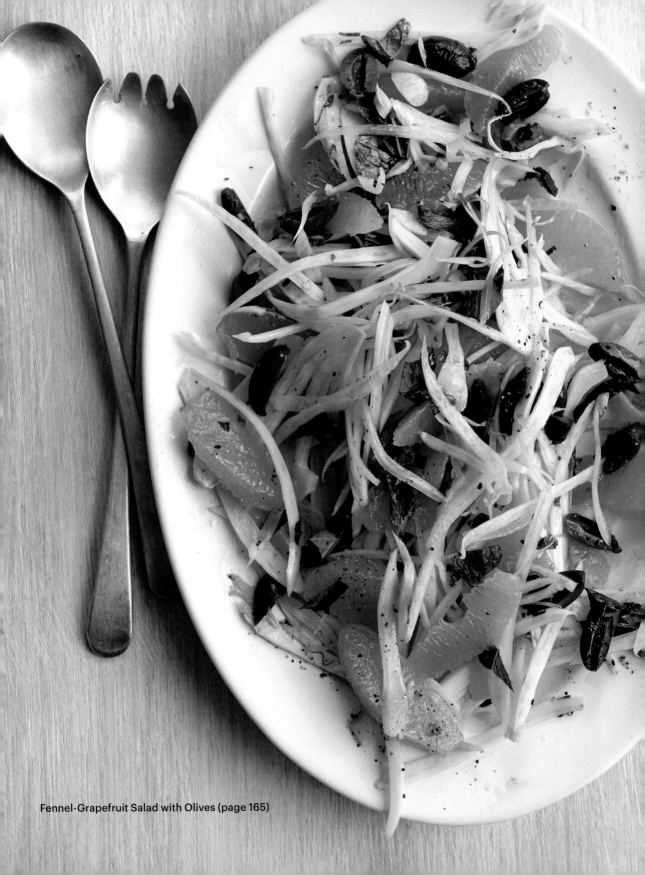

Fennel-Grapefruit Salad with Olives (page 165)

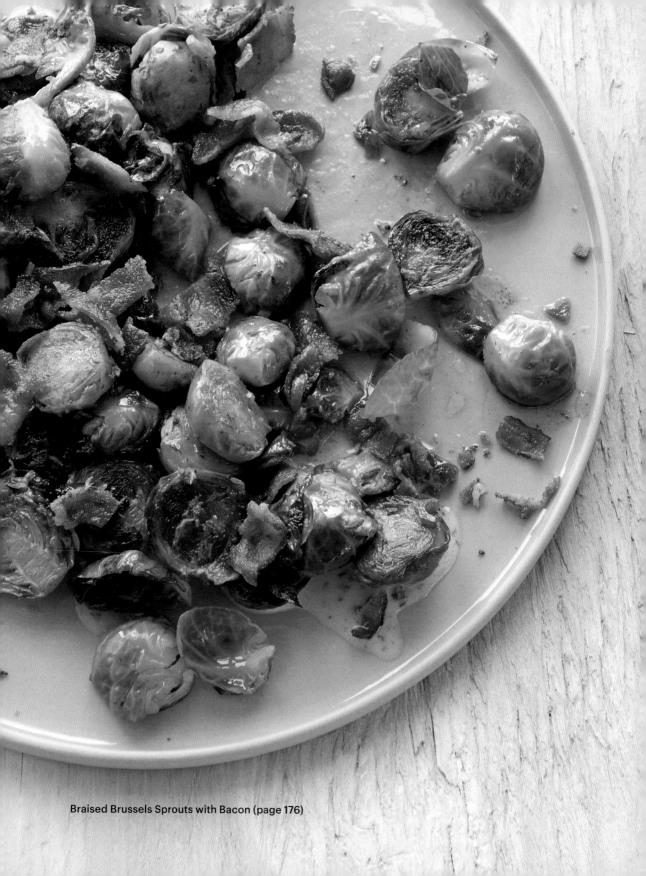

Braised Brussels Sprouts with Bacon (page 176)

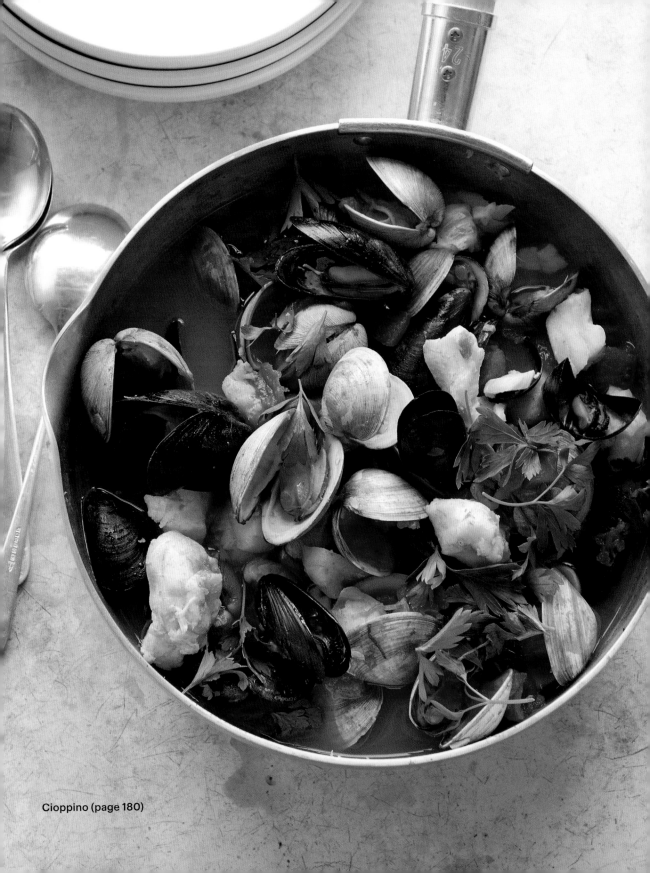

Cioppino (page 180)

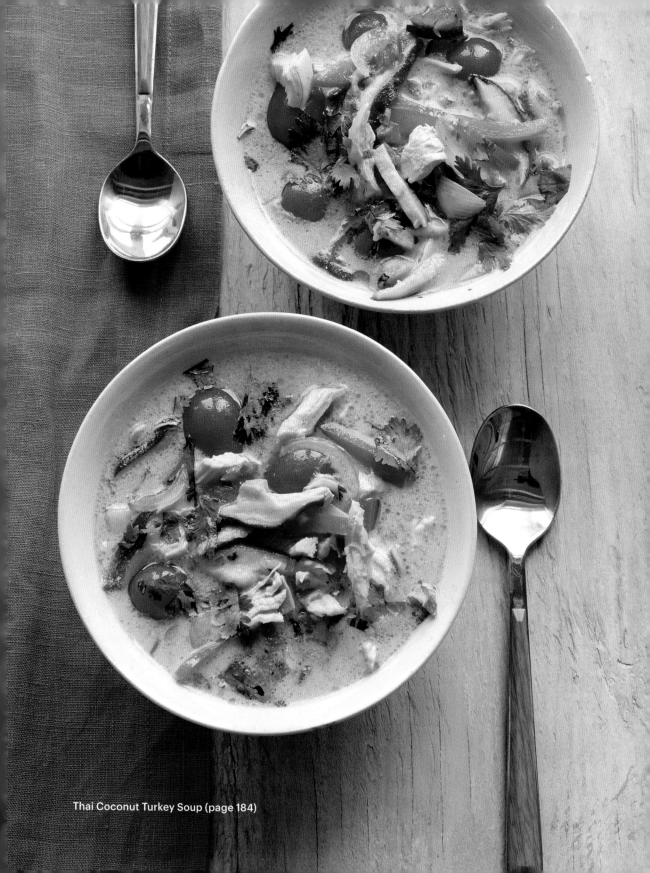

Thai Coconut Turkey Soup (page 184)

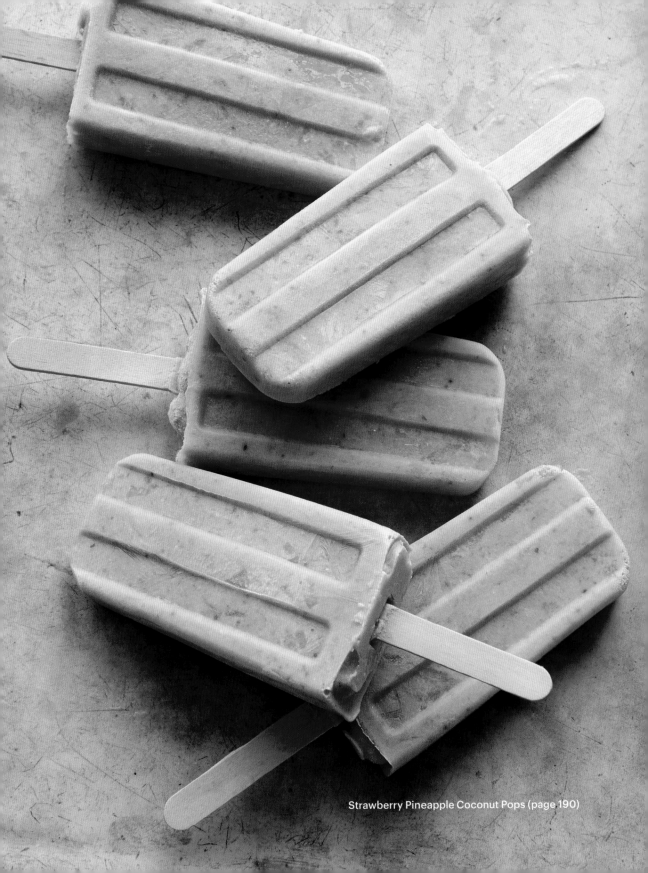

Strawberry Pineapple Coconut Pops (page 190)

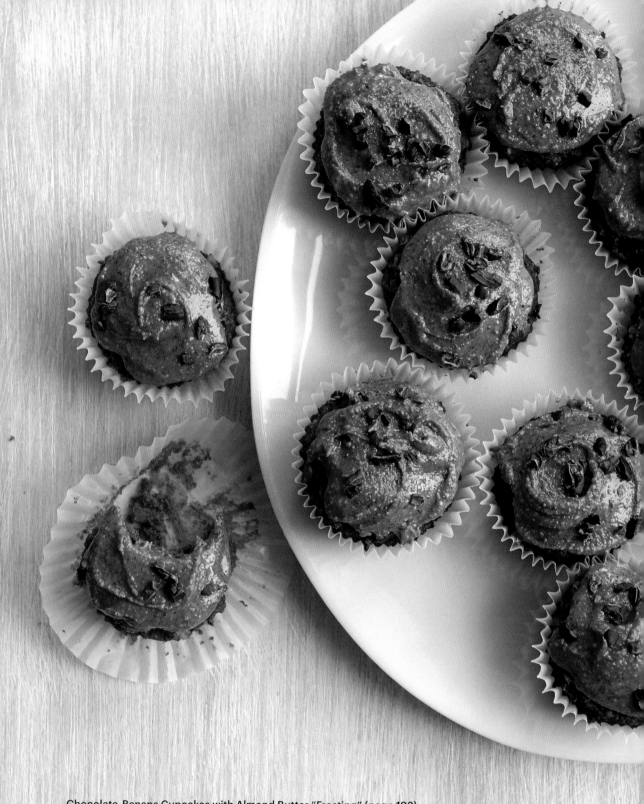

Chocolate-Banana Cupcakes with Almond Butter "Frosting" (page 193)

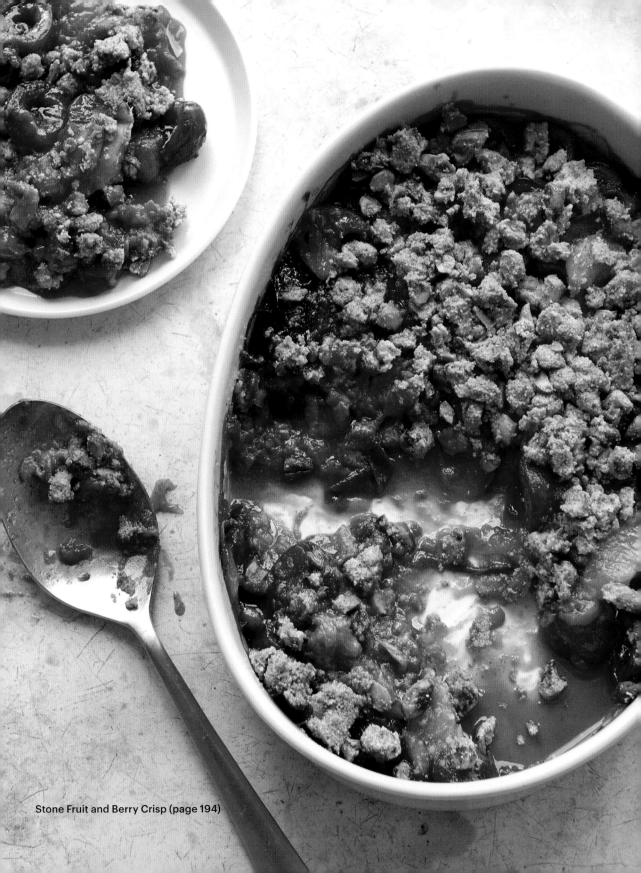

Stone Fruit and Berry Crisp (page 194)

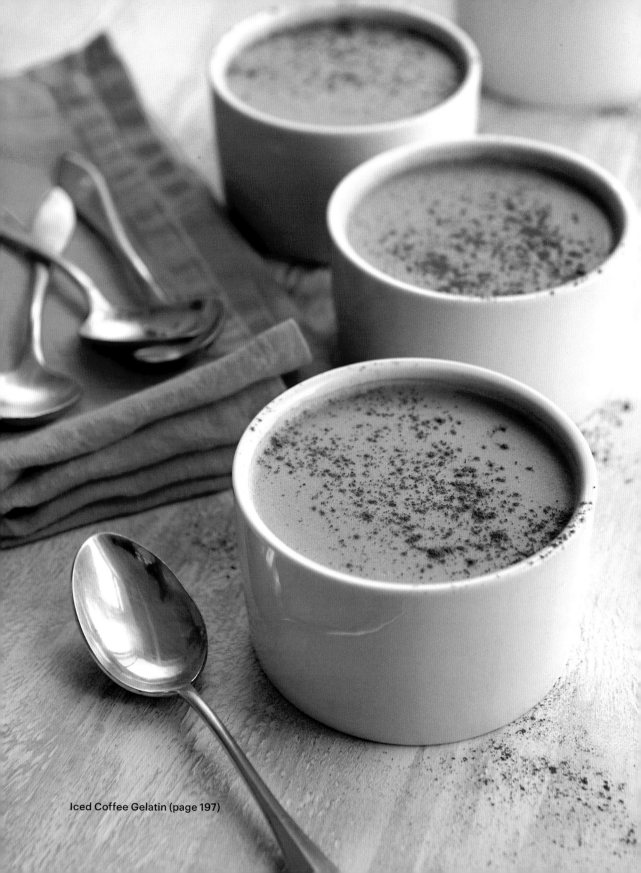

Iced Coffee Gelatin (page 197)

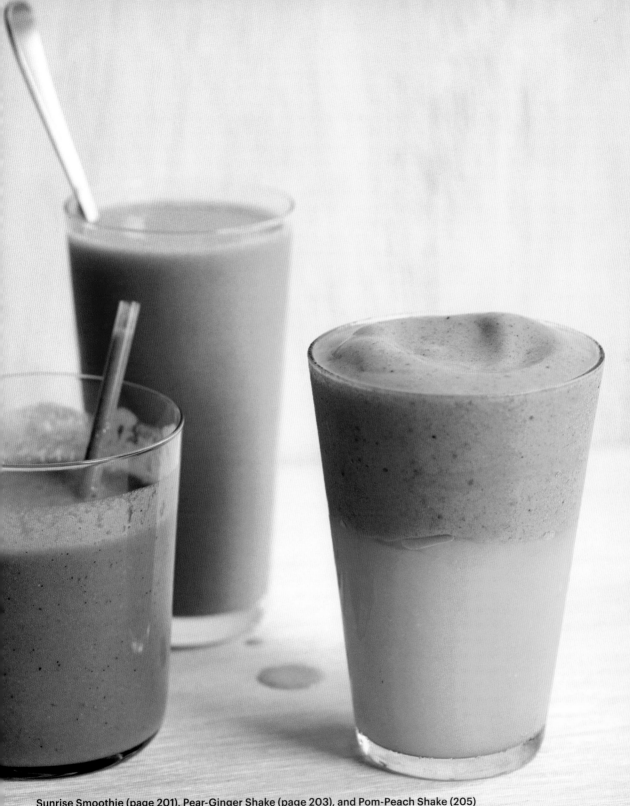

Sunrise Smoothie (page 201), Pear-Ginger Shake (page 203), and Pom-Peach Shake (205)

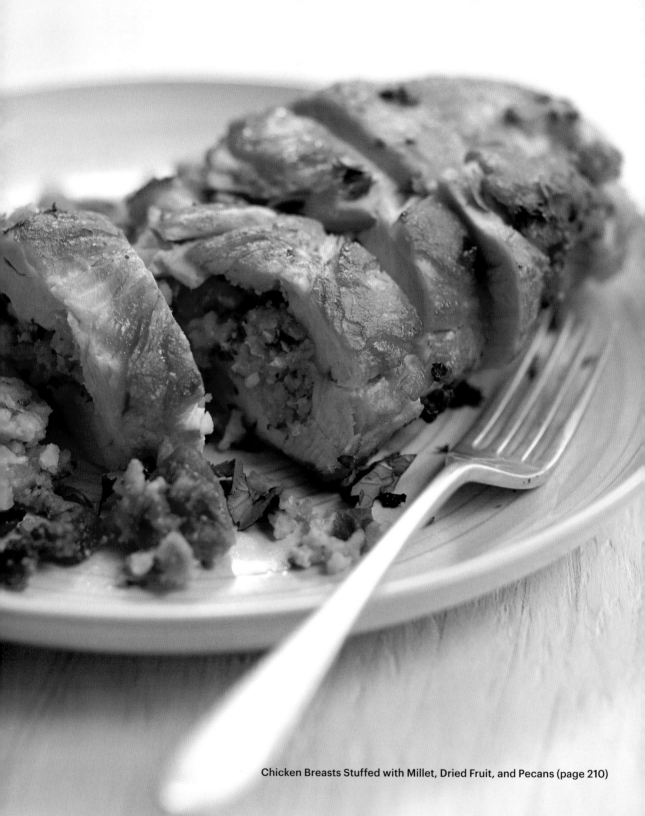

Chicken Breasts Stuffed with Millet, Dried Fruit, and Pecans (page 210)

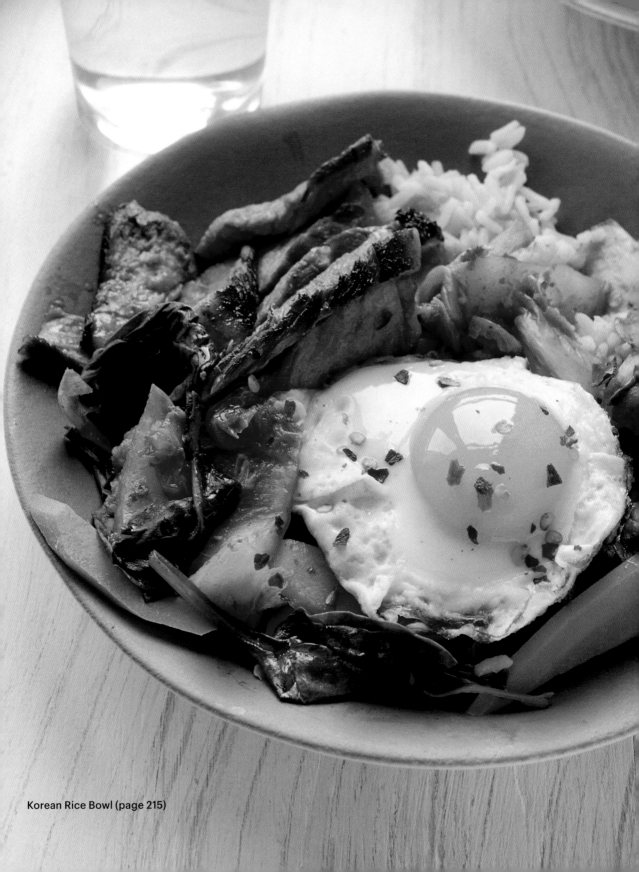

Korean Rice Bowl (page 215)

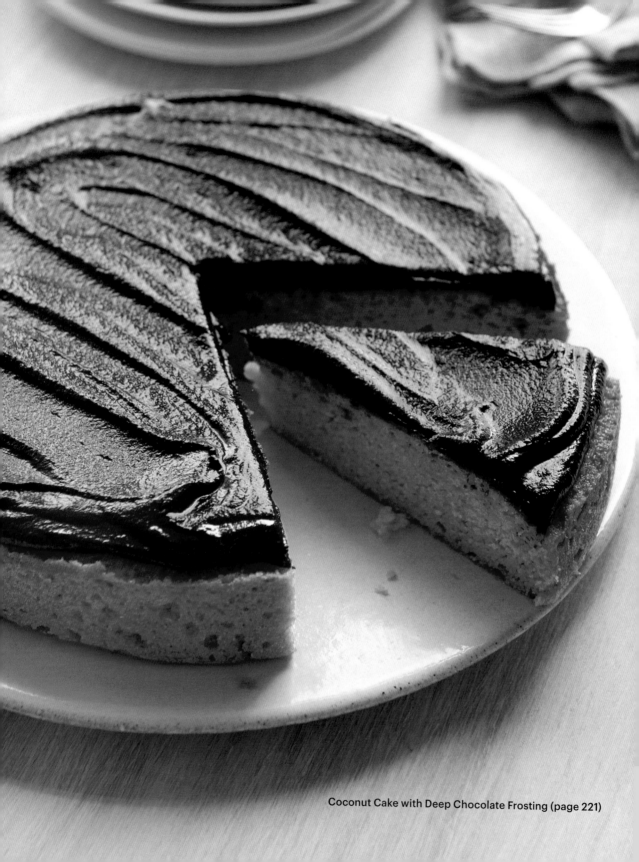

Coconut Cake with Deep Chocolate Frosting (page 221)

# Bliss in a Bowl:
## *Light and Lovely Entree Soups*

IN ITALIAN HOUSEHOLDS LIKE the one I grew up in, life revolves around meals. And these meals, in turn, often revolve around soup—from savory cioppino to spicy meatball soup.

So I've adored soups from an early age. But it wasn't until later that I appreciated the fact that soup—in addition to tasting sensational—is a weight-loss superfood. Here's a look at why it's so terrific.

## SOUP TAKES POUNDS OFF PAINLESSLY

Eating soup before a meal fills you up, so you eat fewer calories. It's much more effective than simply drinking a glass of water before a meal, because water just goes right through you, while soup keeps your stomach full longer.

One study found that people who ate a bowl of soup 15 minutes before lunch ate 20 percent fewer calories overall and felt just as satisfied.[1] Over the course of a year, that can add up to a weight loss of 10 pounds or more . . . with no sacrifice at all!

## SOUP SOOTHES YOUR SOUL

De-stressing is one of the most important things you can do for your health, and it's also crucial if you want to lose weight. That's because stress makes you crave fat and sugar. In addition, it elevates your levels of cortisol, which can add pounds around your waist (I call it a cortisol tire).

Soup made with bone broth is filled with nutrients that calm and relax you, making stress melt away. For instance, it's rich in glycine, which helps to reduce anxiety.

It also gives you a dose of magnesium, a mineral with powerful stress-relieving properties.

When I'm tense and wound up after a long day, I relax with a lovely bowl of soup, like my Gingered Sweet Potato or Thai Coconut Turkey Soup. It relaxes me all over and helps me sleep like a baby—and I know that it's fighting that cortisol tire at the same time.

## FUN WAYS TO "SOUP UP" YOUR DIET

Clearly, it's a good idea to add lots of slimming, stress-reducing soups to your diet. In fact, I recommend having soup nearly every day. Here are three easy, fun ways to do it:

- Start your day with a warm, filling bowl of homemade vegetable beef soup. You'll feel satisfied for hours, and that extra load of veggies will give you a big shot of early-morning nutrition.

- Once or twice a week, pack a thermos of soup for lunch—and bring enough to share with one or two coworkers. They'll appreciate having something far more tasty than their soggy, plastic-packaged meals.

- Once a week, have soup for dinner. Pick a hearty, filling soup, and pair it with a big green salad.

Here's a final tip: Soup is the best way to use up those veggies that are starting to droop in your vegetable bin. Instead of tossing them in the trash, you'll give them new life—and you *and* your wallet will be happy!

# CHUNKY FENNEL-TOMATO SOUP

If you grew up eating tomato soup from a can, you owe it to yourself to taste the real thing. I use fire-roasted tomatoes in this recipe because they have a richer flavor than regular diced tomatoes.

PREP TIME: 10 minutes
COOK TIME: 30 minutes
YIELD: 4 servings
PORTIONS: 1 fat, 2 vegetable

- 3 tablespoons olive oil
- 3 medium yellow or sweet onions, chopped
- 2 medium bulbs fennel, trimmed, cored, and thinly sliced (fronds reserved, if desired)
- 3 cloves garlic, minced
- 1 can (28 ounces) fire-roasted diced tomatoes
- 2 cups Chicken Bone Broth (page 65)
- ¼ teaspoon Celtic or pink Himalayan salt
- ¼ teaspoon freshly ground black pepper
- 4 teaspoons avocado oil

In a large pot, heat the olive oil over medium heat. Add the onions and fennel. Cook, stirring occasionally, until the onions and fennel are golden and tender, about 15 minutes. Add the garlic and cook until fragrant, 1 to 2 minutes. Add the tomatoes with their juice, bone broth, salt, and pepper and bring to a boil. Reduce the heat to medium-low, cover, and simmer until the vegetables are very tender, about 15 minutes more. Season to taste with additional salt and pepper, if necessary.

To serve, divide the soup among 4 bowls and drizzle each with 1 teaspoon avocado oil. Sprinkle with chopped fennel fronds, if using.

**TIPS:**

*Amp up the protein by adding 2 cups shredded cooked chicken to the soup, simmering just until heated through. Or swap out the Chicken Bone Broth and replace with Fish Bone Broth (page 69) and add an 8-ounce can of lump crabmeat, picked over.*

*Chunky's the name of the game for this soup, but if you'd prefer a smoother soup, use an immersion blender to puree the soup until desired consistency. (Alternatively, carefully transfer the soup in batches to a stand blender. Return to the pot to heat through before serving.)*

# CIOPPINO

This traditional Italian fish stew brings clams, mussels, and white fish together in a rich, aromatic broth. A sprinkle of parsley on top adds a colorful touch.

PREP TIME: 10 minutes
COOK TIME: 30 minutes

YIELD: 4 servings

PORTIONS: 1 protein, ½ fat, 1 vegetable

2 tablespoons olive oil

1 large shallot, thinly sliced

2 cloves garlic, minced

¼ teaspoon crushed red-pepper flakes

1 cup Fish Bone Broth (page 69) or store-bought clam juice

1 can (28 ounces) diced tomatoes

1 pound littleneck clams, scrubbed clean

1 pound mussels, scrubbed and debearded (see Tip)

8 ounces flaky white fish, such as cod or haddock, cut into 4 pieces

¼ cup chopped fresh flat-leaf parsley

In a Dutch oven, heat the oil over medium-high heat. Add the shallot, garlic, and pepper flakes and cook, stirring, until the shallot is translucent, about 5 minutes. Stir in the broth and tomatoes with their juice and bring to a boil.

Stir in the clams, cover, and cook for 5 minutes. Add the mussels and fish. Reduce the heat, cover, and cook until the mussels and clams open and the fish flakes easily, about 7 minutes more. Discard any unopened shells and serve sprinkled with parsley.

TIP: *The beard is the mossy-looking bit that hangs off the mussel at the hinge, where the two shells join. It's not inedible, but it is a bit unpleasant. Not every mussel will have a beard, and all it takes is a little tug to pull it free. Tug toward the hinge and give the beard a wiggle to pull it free.*

# GINGERED SWEET POTATO SOUP

Warm up from the inside out with this sweet, subtly Asian-influenced soup. Top it off with avocado, cilantro, and crispy fried garlic to make it picture-perfect.

PREP TIME: 15 minutes

COOK TIME: 25 minutes

YIELD: 4 servings

PORTIONS: 1½ fat, 1 starchy vegetable

¼ cup olive oil

3 cloves garlic: 2 thinly sliced, 1 minced

1 shallot, thinly sliced

1 tablespoon minced fresh ginger

4 cups Asian Chicken Bone Broth (page 72)

2 sweet potatoes (10 to 12 ounces each), peeled and cut into 1-inch chunks (see Tip)

½ cup canned coconut milk, well stirred

Juice of ½ lime

¼ teaspoon Celtic or pink Himalayan salt

¼ teaspoon crushed red-pepper flakes

½ Hass avocado, pitted, peeled, and chopped

2 tablespoons chopped fresh cilantro

In a large pot, heat the oil over medium heat until shimmering. Add half of the sliced garlic and fry until the edges are golden, 45 to 60 seconds. Remove with a slotted spoon to a paper towel. Repeat with the remaining sliced garlic.

Pour out all but 1 tablespoon of the oil from the pot and return the pot to medium heat. Add the shallot, ginger, and minced garlic and cook, stirring frequently, until softened, 5 minutes. Add the broth and sweet potatoes and bring to a boil. Reduce the heat to medium-low and simmer, partially covered, until the potatoes are tender when pierced with a knife, 15 to 20 minutes.

With an immersion blender, puree the soup until smooth. (Alternatively, carefully transfer in batches to a stand blender, then return to the pot.) Stir in the coconut milk, lime juice, salt, and pepper flakes. Heat through and taste to adjust for seasoning, if necessary.

To serve, divide the soup among 4 bowls. Top each serving with avocado, cilantro, and crispy fried garlic.

TIP: *Peeled butternut squash makes a delicious substitute for sweet potatoes.*

# BUTTERNUT SQUASH and CHICKEN APPLE SAUSAGE SOUP

This thick, hearty, sage-scented soup is topped with bite-size bits of sausage. It's one of my favorite comfort foods on a cold, rainy day.

PREP TIME: 10 minutes

COOK TIME: 30 minutes

YIELD: 6 servings

PORTIONS: ½ protein, ½ fat, 1 starchy vegetable

3 tablespoons coconut oil

2½ pounds butternut squash, peeled, seeded, and cut into 1-inch chunks

1 medium onion, chopped

1½ tablespoons finely chopped fresh sage

Celtic or pink Himalayan salt and freshly ground black pepper

4 cups Chicken Bone Broth (page 65)

1 tablespoon apple cider vinegar

3 chicken apple sausage links, chopped

In a 5-quart saucepan, heat 2 tablespoons of the coconut oil over medium heat until shimmering. Add the squash, onion, and sage and cook until lightly browned, about 8 minutes. Season generously with salt and pepper. Add the broth, scraping up any browned bits on the bottom with a wooden spoon.

Bring to a boil, then reduce to a simmer and cook until the squash is very soft, about 10 minutes. Remove from the heat and let cool slightly. With an immersion blender, puree the soup until smooth. (Alternatively, carefully transfer in batches to a stand blender. Return to the saucepan.) Stir in the apple cider vinegar and season to taste with additional salt and pepper.

Meanwhile, in a small skillet, heat the remaining 1 tablespoon oil over medium heat. Add the sausage and cook until lightly browned and crisped, about 5 minutes.

Serve the soup with the chicken sausage sprinkled on top.

# SPICY MEATBALL SOUP

Smoked paprika and cayenne pepper give this soup an extra kick. You can make the meatballs on your batch cooking day and then freeze them to use later.

PREP TIME: 15 minutes

COOK TIME: 25 minutes

YIELD: 4 servings

PORTIONS: ½ protein, ¼ fat, ¼ vegetable

½ pound ground meat (turkey, chicken, or beef)

1 large egg

1 tablespoon chopped fresh flat-leaf parsley

Celtic or pink Himalayan salt and freshly ground black pepper

Pinch of cayenne pepper

1 tablespoon olive oil

1 medium onion, chopped

1 green bell pepper, chopped

6 cups Beef Bone Broth (page 67)

1 can (14.5 ounces) fire-roasted diced tomatoes

½ teaspoon smoked paprika

In a medium bowl, mix together the meat, egg, parsley, ¼ teaspoon salt, ¼ teaspoon pepper, and cayenne. Form into 18 one-inch balls and set aside.

In a large pot, heat the oil over medium heat. Add the onion and bell pepper and cook until softened, about 5 minutes. Add the broth, tomatoes and their juice, and smoked paprika and bring to a simmer. Add the meatballs, stir gently, and cook until no longer pink inside, about 20 minutes. Season to taste with salt and pepper.

# THAI COCONUT TURKEY SOUP

A cornucopia of yummy veggies makes every bite of this soup delicious. Garnish with a generous sprinkling of cilantro and, if you like it hot, some sliced Thai bird chile.

PREP TIME: 10 minutes

COOK TIME: 25 minutes

YIELD: 4 servings

PORTIONS: ¼ protein, 1 fat, ¼ vegetable

2 tablespoons coconut oil

1 medium yellow onion, thinly sliced

1 medium red bell pepper, thinly sliced

12 ounces sliced shiitake mushroom caps

1 tablespoon minced fresh ginger

1 tablespoon minced garlic

1 cup cherry tomatoes

4 cups Thanksgiving Turkey Bone Broth (page 70)

½ cup canned coconut milk, well stirred

1 tablespoon Thai green curry paste

1 cup shredded cooked turkey meat

Celtic or pink Himalayan salt

¼ cup chopped fresh cilantro

1 fresh red Thai bird chile (optional), thinly sliced (wear gloves when handling)

In a 4-quart saucepan, melt the coconut oil over medium heat. Add the onion and bell pepper and cook until they begin to soften, about 5 minutes. Add the mushrooms, ginger, and garlic and cook until the mushrooms are soft and begin to release their liquid, about 5 minutes. Add the tomatoes and cook until their skins begin to soften, about 3 minutes.

In a bowl, whisk together the broth, coconut milk, and curry paste until the curry paste is incorporated. Add the mixture to the saucepan and bring to a simmer. Add the shredded turkey and cook until the turkey is heated through, about 2 minutes. Season to taste with salt.

To serve, divide among 4 wide shallow bowls and garnish with the cilantro and chile (if using).

# GREEN SOUP

This is a great go-to soup when you're in a hurry and want a big surge of energy! And if anyone in your family is under the weather, this is the very best medicine.

PREP TIME: 15 minutes

COOK TIME: 15 minutes

YIELD: 4 servings

PORTION: 1 vegetable

4–6 cups Chicken Bone Broth (page 65) or chicken stock

¼ teaspoon ground turmeric

3 cloves garlic, thinly sliced

1–2 large leeks, white parts only, washed thoroughly and thinly sliced

3 heads baby bok choy, each cut into 6–8 wedges

¼ teaspoon Celtic or pink Himalayan salt

Freshly ground black pepper

In a 2-quart pot, bring the broth to a simmer over medium heat. Add the turmeric, garlic, and leeks and simmer for 10 minutes. Add the bok choy and season with salt and pepper; stir. Simmer for about 2 minutes more. Once the bok choy is tender and bright green, serve immediately.

*Recipe developed and written by Karen Pickus*
*Courtesy Karen Pickus 2016*

# CHILLED GREEN POWER SOUP

This chilled soup is fantastic on a hot summer day. It doesn't require any cooking, and it revs you up when the heat of the day has you wilting.

PREP TIME: 15 to 20 minutes

YIELD: 4 servings

PORTIONS: 1 fat, 1 vegetable

1 red bell pepper, half finely chopped and half cut into chunks

1 European cucumber, half finely chopped and half cut into chunks

1 lemon, zested, then peeled and segmented

½ ripe avocado, cut into chunks

1 cup baby spinach

1 cup baby kale

⅔ cup fresh flat-leaf parsley leaves

1 clove garlic, peeled

1 cup canned coconut milk, lightly stirred

½ cup water

6 ice cubes

⅛ teaspoon Celtic or pink Himalayan salt

⅛ teaspoon cayenne pepper (optional)

In a small bowl, combine the finely chopped red pepper, finely chopped cucumber, and lemon zest; set aside.

In a blender, combine the red pepper chunks, cucumber chunks, avocado chunks, lemon juice, spinach, kale, parsley, garlic, coconut milk, water, ice cubes, salt, and cayenne (if using). Puree until smooth. You may need to stop the blender a few times and move the ingredients along with the handle of a wooden spoon.

To serve, divide among 4 soup bowls and top with the garnish.

*Recipe developed and written by Karen Pickus*
*Courtesy Karen Pickus 2016*

# APPLE-CUCUMBER-LIME CHILLED SUMMER SOUP

This is a perfect starter for supper on a hot evening. It's quick and easy: Just chop, zest, blend, and go!

PREP TIME: 15 to 20 minutes

YIELD: 4 servings

PORTIONS: ¼ fat, 1 fruit

2 green apples, 1½ cut into 2-inch chunks and ½ finely chopped

1 European cucumber, ⅔ cut into 2-inch chunks and ⅓ finely chopped

Grated peel and juice of 1 lime

1 tablespoon grated fresh ginger

4 ice cubes

½ cup canned coconut milk, lightly stirred

In a bowl, combine the finely chopped apples, finely chopped cucumber, and lime peel; set aside.

In a blender, combine the apple chunks, cucumber chunks, lime juice, ginger, ice cubes, and coconut milk. Puree until very smooth.

Serve immediately, topped with the garnish.

*Recipe developed and written by Karen Pickus*
*Courtesy Karen Pickus 2016*

## CHAPTER 10

# A Little Something Sweet:

## *Yummy Desserts That Are Guilt-Free—Really!*

**NOTHING MAKES A NICER** end to a meal than something sweet—and yes, you *can* have delicious sweet treats on my diet! In fact, in this chapter, you'll find recipes for everything from sorbet and popsicles to cupcakes and fresh berry crisp.

Now, I suspect that you may be wondering, "How can you make dessert without sugar or other sweeteners?" The answer is simple: by incorporating *fruit*. Fruit is one of the world's original sweeteners, and it's still the very best one.

However, there's something I want you to know: If you're used to gooey dough-nuts and sugary cupcakes, fruit desserts initially might not seem sweet enough. For a little while when you start my diet, you may still find yourself craving sugar-loaded brownies, ice cream, and cookies.

Biologically, there's a good reason for this. Here's the story about why sugar has a powerful hold over you, and how my delicious desserts can help you break that spell.

## WHY SUGAR HAS ITS HOOKS IN YOU

Food cravings originate in our brains—and millions of years ago, those cravings made perfect sense. Back then, the only sweet foods available were fruits and honey, and each provided a hefty dose of nutrients, along with a little bit of sugar.

Because sweets were both scarce and nutritious back then, our genes learned a big lesson: *Sweet is good.* As a result, those genes programmed our body chemistry to make us crave sugary foods. This craving worked just fine for thousands of years. But then came packaged and processed foods, and that's when our epic battle with the Sugar Demon began.

You see, that message our genes programmed into us — *sweet food is good* — works only when sweet foods are both nutrient-dense and scarce. But in a world of processed foods, there's no brake on our craving for sweets. The more we get, the more we want — and today, the supply of sugary junk food is endless.

Worse yet, manufacturers have altered our tastebuds in ways that make us walk right past the fruit aisle and head for the cookie aisle instead. They've done this by loading their desserts with far more sugar than natural fruit contains. Over time, this makes our tastebuds become hyporesponsive to sugar, meaning that an apple or a handful of berries might not give us the sugar "hit" we're craving.

## PUT THE SUGAR DEMON BACK IN HIS PLACE

Because your tastebuds are trained to expect a huge hit of sugar, the best way to conquer the Sugar Demon is to *retrain* them. And luckily, it won't take as long as you might think.

The first step, which you're taking right now if you're doing my diet, is to cut out sugar and artificial sweeteners entirely. The next step is to recalibrate your tastebuds — and here's how to do it.

Each time you eat one of my fruit desserts, savor the first few bites very, very, *very* slowly. (You can also do this with a piece of fruit or a sweet red bell pepper.) Allow your tastebuds to seek out the sugar and appreciate it. Let the food rest on your tongue for a little while. Really get into the "zen" of this.

Over time, a surprising thing will happen: Your little treat will suddenly start to "pop" with sweetness. That's because you're waking up your tastebuds, and they're rediscovering the joy of eating naturally sweet foods. And eventually, you'll discover something even *more* surprising: Those grocery-store sweets are going to taste cloyingly sweet and artificial, and you'll wonder what you ever saw in them.

In short, the recipes in this chapter won't just provide a delicious ending to a meal, they'll also teach your tastebuds to love healthy desserts, and they'll help you slay the Sugar Demon forever. How's *that* for sweet?

# STRAWBERRY PINEAPPLE COCONUT POPS

In these sweet treats, bites of pineapple are tucked into a mix of pureed strawberries and creamy coconut milk. Kids love them—and so do grown-ups!

PREP TIME: 10 minutes
FREEZE TIME: 5 to 7 hours
YIELD: 10 servings
PORTIONS: ¼ fat, ¾ fruit

2½ cups hulled strawberries

1 can (14.5 ounces) coconut milk

1 cup finely chopped fresh pineapple

In a blender or food processor, puree the strawberries. Transfer to a large measuring cup or bowl with a pouring spout and stir in the coconut milk.

Divide the pineapple among ten ⅓-cup ice pop molds. Pour in the strawberry mixture, leaving ¼ inch at the top to allow for expansion. Stir each mold gently with an ice pop stick to get the pineapple pieces floating in the strawberry mixture. Freeze for about 1 hour, then insert the ice pop sticks. Return to the freezer until fully set, another 4 to 6 hours.

To unmold, let the pops sit at room temperature until they easily slide out, about 5 minutes. Wrap each pop individually in plastic wrap and store in the freezer. The pops taste best if eaten within 3 weeks.

# APPLE POMEGRANATE COMPOTE

Apples and figs simmer in spiced apple juice until they're syrupy, then get a crunchy topping of chopped pistachios and pomegranate seeds.

PREP TIME: 5 minutes

COOK TIME: 40 minutes

YIELD: 6 servings

PORTIONS: ½ fat, 1 fruit

- 1 cup unsweetened apple juice
- 2 whole cloves
- 1 star anise
- 1 cinnamon stick
- 2 apples, peeled, cored, and chopped
- ½ cup dried figs, chopped
- 6 tablespoons pistachios, chopped
- 6 tablespoons pomegranate seeds (arils)

In a medium saucepan, combine the apple juice, cloves, star anise, cinnamon stick, apples, and figs. Bring to a boil over medium heat, reduce the heat to low, and simmer until reduced and syrupy, 35 to 40 minutes. Remove and discard the whole spices.

To serve, divide the mixture among 4 small bowls. Top with the pistachios and pomegranate seeds and serve.

## MAKE IT A 20

*Serve over amaranth cooked in almond milk for a warming porridge.*

# FRUITY GELATIN

Forget that sugary, artificially-flavored stuff in a box! It's fun and easy to make your own gelatin from scratch.

PREP TIME: 5 minutes

COOK TIME: 10 minutes plus chilling time

YIELD: 6 servings

PORTION: 1 fruit

2½ cups unsweetened apple juice or unfiltered unsweetened apple cider

1 tablespoon unflavored pasture-raised beef gelatin, such as Great Lakes Gelatin (see Tips)

½ cup cubed apple, halved grapes, or blackberries (see Tips)

Pour ½ cup of the juice in a shallow bowl. Sprinkle the gelatin evenly over the surface and set aside until the gelatin is no longer powdery and the juice is gelatinous, about 10 minutes. (If it still looks powdery, gently stir to combine.)

Meanwhile, in a medium saucepan, bring the remaining 2 cups juice to a simmer over medium heat; do not boil. Remove from the heat.

Slowly add the gelatin mixture to the hot juice, stirring to fully dissolve the gelatin. Pour the liquid into an 8 × 8-inch glass baking dish or other shallow glass container and refrigerate until slightly set (not entirely liquid), about 1 hour. Stir in the fruit, then return to the refrigerator until completely set, 1 to 2 hours more.

Scoop and serve (see Tips). Store any remaining gelatin in a covered container for up to 1 week.

**TIPS:**

*This recipe works with almost any fruit juice—or fruit-vegetable combination—but avoid kiwifruit, mango, guava, fig, pineapple, or papaya, as they contain enzymes that will prevent the gelatin from setting up. If you have a juicer, all the better to make exotic combinations.*

*To make more solid blocks of gelatin, add another tablespoon of gelatin to the cool juice before mixing into the hot juice.*

*A fun serving idea is to present these as cubes. Pour the finished liquid mixture into silicone ice cube trays and dot with bits of fruit and mint leaves.*

# CHOCOLATE-BANANA CUPCAKES with ALMOND BUTTER "FROSTING"

Craving chocolate? Then whip up a batch of these cupcakes that promise a double dose: cocoa powder in the batter and cacao nibs sprinkled over the frosting.

PREP TIME: 10 minutes
COOK TIME: 30 minutes plus cooling time
YIELD: 24 servings
PORTIONS: 1½ fat, ¼ fruit

- 1¼ cups almond flour
- 2 tablespoons coconut flour
- 2 tablespoons ground flaxseeds
- 2 tablespoons unsweetened cocoa powder
- 1½ teaspoons baking powder
- ½ teaspoon ground cinnamon
- ¼ teaspoon Celtic or pink Himalayan salt
- 3 ripe medium bananas, mashed
- ⅓ cup coconut oil, melted and cooled
- 2 large eggs
- 2½ teaspoons vanilla extract
- ¾ cup natural almond butter
- 1 tablespoon cacao nibs
- 2 teaspoons flaky Celtic or pink Himalayan salt

Preheat the oven to 350°F. Line 24 cups of a mini muffin pan with paper liners and coat the liners with coconut oil spray.

In a large bowl, whisk together the almond flour, coconut flour, ground flax, cocoa, baking powder, cinnamon, and salt.

In a medium bowl, combine the bananas, coconut oil, eggs, and 1 teaspoon of the vanilla and stir until smooth. Add the banana mixture to the flour mixture and stir just until blended.

Divide the batter among the muffin cups and bake until a wooden pick inserted into the center of a cupcake comes out clean, about 15 minutes. Cool in the pan on a rack for 5 minutes. Remove and cool completely before frosting.

In a small bowl, with an electric mixer, whip the almond butter and remaining 1½ teaspoons vanilla until light and smooth. Spread over the cooled cupcakes. Sprinkle cacao nibs and some flaky salt over the cupcakes before serving.

# STONE FRUIT and BERRY CRISP

Apricots, plums, raspberries, and cherries come together in this simple crisp, topped off with an almond crumble. Arrowroot gives the filling a lovely texture.

PREP TIME: 15 minutes

COOK TIME: 45 minutes

YIELD: 9 servings

PORTIONS: 1 fat, 1 fruit

½ cup almond flour

½ cup pistachios, coarsely chopped

½ teaspoon ground cinnamon

Celtic or pink Himalayan salt

2 tablespoons coconut oil

2 apricots, pitted and sliced

1 plum, pitted and sliced

1 cup raspberries

½ cup cherries, pitted and halved

1 tablespoon arrowroot powder

Preheat the oven to 350°F. Grease an 8 × 8-inch baking pan or small casserole dish with coconut oil and set aside.

In a small bowl, combine the almond flour, pistachios, cinnamon, and a pinch of salt. Using a fork or your fingers, cut in the coconut oil until the mixture resembles wet sand.

In a large bowl, stir together the apricots, plum, raspberries, cherries, arrowroot powder, and a pinch of salt. Pour into the prepared pan and top with the almond flour mixture. Bake, uncovered, until bubbling, 30 to 35 minutes. Cool for 15 minutes and cut into 9 portions before serving.

Serve warm or cold, and store any remaining crisp in the refrigerator.

TIP: *This crisp will taste best with the freshest in-season fruit you can find!*

# GINGER-POACHED ASIAN PEARS with COCONUT-CARDAMOM CREAM

These pears simmer gently in a vanilla-and-spice bath. Once tender, drizzle them with syrup and top with a dollop of coconut-cardamom cream.

PREP TIME: 5 minutes
COOK TIME: 45 minutes
YIELD: 4 servings
PORTIONS: ¼ fat, 1 fruit

- 8 slices fresh ginger (each ⅛-inch thick)
- 8 whole cloves
- 2 cardamom pods
- 1 cinnamon stick
- 1 star anise
- ½ vanilla bean
- 2 Asian pears, halved, peeled, and cored
- ⅓ cup coconut cream (see Tip)
- ¼ teaspoon ground cardamom
- ⅛ teaspoon ground ginger

In a medium saucepan, combine 3 cups water, fresh ginger, cloves, cardamom pods, cinnamon stick, and star anise. Split the vanilla beans, scrape the seeds into the pan, and then throw in the vanilla pod. Bring to a boil, reduce the heat to medium-low, and add the pears. Cover and simmer, turning the pears occasionally, until a paring knife slides easily into the thickest portion, 25 to 30 minutes.

Remove the pears to a dish and cover with foil. Strain the spices out of the poaching liquid and return the liquid to the pan. Bring to a gentle boil over medium-high heat and cook until the syrup is reduced to ½ cup, about 20 minutes.

Meanwhile, in a medium bowl, with an electric mixer or a whisk, beat the coconut cream, ground cardamom, and ground ginger until thick.

To serve, spoon the syrup over the pears and dollop with the spiced cream.

**TIP:** *Coconut cream is available wherever canned coconut milk is sold. If you can't find it, chill a can of regular full-fat coconut milk and scoop out the solid white part that solidifies at the top.*

### MAKE IT A 20
*Add 2 tablespoons maple syrup to the liquid while the pears poach.*

# MANGO-LIME SORBET

The trick to this yummy sorbet is to make sure your mangoes are very ripe and supersweet. The rest is easy—just blend your ingredients and pop them into an ice cream maker, and you're done.

PREP TIME: 10 minutes

COOK TIME: 5 minutes plus freezing time

YIELD: 5 to 6 servings (about 1 pint)

PORTION: 1 fruit

2 very ripe mangoes, pitted and peeled

Grated peel and juice of 1 lime

½ cup fresh orange juice

¼ teaspoon Celtic or pink Himalayan salt

In a food processor or blender, combine the mangoes, lime peel, lime juice, orange juice, and salt. Process or blend until very smooth. Pour the mixture into an ice cream maker and freeze according to the manufacturer's instructions. Transfer to an airtight container and store in the freezer until ready to use, up to 1 month.

# ICED COFFEE GELATIN

I love this light, refreshing after-dinner treat. It's coffee and dessert in one shot!

PREP TIME: 5 minutes
COOK TIME: 1 hour
YIELD: 4 servings
PORTION: ½ fat

- 1 cup canned coconut milk, well stirred
- 2 tablespoons unflavored pasture-raised beef gelatin (such as Great Lakes Gelatin)
- 2 cups hot brewed coffee
- 1 teaspoon vanilla extract

Pour the coconut milk into a medium bowl. Sprinkle the gelatin over the coconut milk and let rest for 1 minute, then whisk the gelatin into the coconut milk. Add the hot coffee and vanilla and whisk until the gelatin is completely dissolved, about 2 minutes.

Pour into an 8 × 8-inch pan (or four ½-cup ramekins), cover, and refrigerate until firm, 1 hour or more.

## MAKE IT A 20

*Stir in 2 tablespoons maple syrup with the hot coffee.*

# ALOHA BOWL

Take a trip to Hawaii without leaving your kitchen. This cool, creamy, soft-serve dessert features bananas, pineapple, mango, coconut chips, and macadamia nuts—all in one bowl.

PREP TIME: 5 minutes
COOK TIME: 5 minutes

YIELD: 4 servings

PORTIONS: 1 fat, 1 fruit

¾ cup frozen banana chunks

¾ cup frozen pineapple chunks

½ cup frozen mango chunks

½ cup unsweetened almond milk

¼ cup macadamia nuts, toasted and coarsely chopped

¼ cup toasted coconut chips

1 tablespoon cacao nibs

1 tablespoon bee pollen

In a blender, combine the banana, pineapple, mango, and almond milk and blend until the mixture reaches a thick, soft-serve consistency. Divide among 4 chilled bowls and top each with nuts, coconut chips, cacao nibs, and bee pollen. Serve immediately.

## CHAPTER 11

# Meals in Minutes:

## *Quick Shakes and Smoothies for Wild-and-Crazy Days*

MORNINGS AROUND MY HOUSE are absolute chaos. I hit the ground running as soon as the alarm goes off, and I still barely make it out the door on time. Something always comes up—whether it's a phone call, a run in my panty hose, or one of my boys saying, "Mom! I can't find my jacket!"

If your mornings are just as crazy as mine, you may not have time to scramble eggs or even heat up leftovers. Luckily, I have a simple solution: Shake it up.

You can prepare a shake or smoothie in just minutes—or even seconds, if you prep your ingredients ahead of time (see page 51). And while these luscious drinks are super speedy, they're also packed with nutrition that will keep you going for hours.

By the way, if you're wondering what the difference is between shakes and smoothies, the answer is: very little. I use the term *shakes* for drinks that replace milk with protein powder, almond milk, or sometimes coconut kefir. My smoothies, on the other hand, simply contain fruits and sometimes vegetables. But you can call these delicious drinks by any name you like, as long as you enjoy them!

### WHY NOT WHEY?

Many people think that whey is fine on a dairy-free diet because it doesn't contain casein, the milk protein that's most likely to cause sensitivity. However, casein is only part of the story. Some whey protein powders contain significant amounts of the milk sugar lactose, which can cause gas, bloating, and diarrhea. Others are nearly or entirely lactose-free but can still cause GI problems because many people are sensitive to whey itself.

Beef protein gives you the high-quality nutrition you want without exposing you to lactose or whey. As a result, you get all the benefits of a protein supplement, without the potential drawbacks. Just make sure you select a beef protein supplement that's derived from grass-fed animals (like mine, which you can obtain at drkellyannstore.com) to ensure that you're getting the highest quality of protein.

## TIPS FOR SHAKES

My shake and smoothie recipes are fabulous—but feel free to improvise and create your own, as long as you stick to my approved foods. Here are some fun ways to change things up:

- You can add a serving of fat to your drink by adding 1 teaspoon coconut oil.

- You can add more creaminess and a fat serving with half an avocado. Avocado doesn't change the flavor, making it an ideal fat to add to any shake.

- Want to get some additional healthy greens in your diet? Then add 1 cup tightly packed fresh spinach. Believe it or not, spinach won't add any flavor to your shake, although it *will* turn it green.

- You can make your drinks creamier by using frozen fruit or adding a couple of ice cubes.

- For variety, add chia seeds or ground flaxseeds to your shake or smoothie. Count each tablespoon as half a fat serving.

Shakes and smoothies are also an outstanding way to take advantage of seasonal produce. Buying fruits and vegetables in season is the best way to get a good price and maximum nutrition, so feel free to swap out my ingredients for the specials at your local farmers' market. I've invented some of my own favorite recipes that way!

# SUNRISE SMOOTHIE

Like a sunrise, this smoothie has beautiful layers of orange and red. It features yummy mango and strawberries.

PREP TIME: 10 minutes

YIELD: 2 servings

PORTIONS: 1 protein, 1 fruit

**For the orange layer:**

- ½ cup mango chunks, frozen
- ½ cup cold water
- 1 scoop vanilla SLIM Protein or Dr. Kellyann–approved protein powder

**For the red layer:**

- ½ cup frozen sliced strawberries
- ½ cup water
- ¼ cup ice cubes
- 1 scoop vanilla SLIM Protein or Dr. Kellyann–approved protein powder

*For the orange layer*: In a blender, puree the mango, water, and protein powder. Transfer to a measuring cup and rinse the blender.

*For the red layer*: Puree the strawberries, water, ice, and protein powder.

Divide between 2 glasses, alternating between the orange and red mixtures to create a beautiful sunrise in your glass.

# PUMPKIN PIE SHAKE

This shake delivers all of the flavors of pumpkin pie—and it's sin-free! Be sure to use pumpkin puree rather than pumpkin pie filling.

PREP TIME: 10 minutes

YIELD: 2 servings

PORTIONS: 1 protein, ½ fat, 1 fruit, 1 starchy vegetable

- 2 cups unsweetened almond milk
- ½ ripe banana
- ½ cup canned unsweetened pumpkin puree
- ½ cup ice cubes
- 2 scoops vanilla SLIM Protein or Dr. Kellyann–approved protein powder
- 1 tablespoon natural almond butter
- 2 pitted dates
- ½ teaspoon pumpkin pie spice
- Ground cinnamon, for serving

In a blender, puree the almond milk, banana, pumpkin puree, ice, protein powder, almond butter, dates, and pumpkin pie spice. Divide between 2 glasses and sprinkle with cinnamon.

# PEAR-GINGER SHAKE

The spinach in this shake adds a burst of nutrition—and you won't even taste it. It's a great way to help kids eat an extra serving of vegetables.

PREP TIME: 5 minutes

YIELD: 2 servings

PORTIONS: 1 protein, 1 fruit, 1 vegetable

1 pear, cored and chopped

2 cups baby spinach

1½ cups unsweetened almond milk

2 scoops vanilla SLIM Protein or Dr. Kellyann–approved protein powder

2 teaspoons fresh lemon juice

1 teaspoon grated fresh ginger

½ teaspoon vanilla extract

⅛ teaspoon ground nutmeg

In a blender, puree the pear, spinach, almond milk, protein powder, lemon juice, ginger, vanilla, and nutmeg until smooth and frothy, about 1 minute.

# ICY MOCHA KEFIR SHAKE

If you're a coffee lover, you'll be in heaven when you taste this. The banana adds sweetness, while the cocoa powder provides a hit of chocolate.

PREP TIME: 5 minutes

YIELD: 2 servings

PORTIONS: ½ protein, ½ fat, ½ fruit

1 cup unsweetened plain coconut-milk kefir

½ banana, frozen

¼ cup brewed espresso or strong coffee, cooled

1 scoop chocolate SLIM Protein or Dr. Kellyann–approved protein powder

1 teaspoon unsweetened cocoa powder

¼ teaspoon vanilla extract

½ cup ice cubes

In a blender, puree the kefir, banana, espresso, protein powder, cocoa, vanilla, and ice until creamy and frothy, about 1 minute.

# POM-PEACH SHAKE

Pomegranate juice, peaches, and raspberries blend to make a light, refreshing shake that's perfect for breakfast or an afternoon pick-me-up. And it's not just delicious—it's *loaded* with antioxidant power.

PREP TIME: 3 minutes

YIELD: 2 servings

PORTIONS: ½ protein, ½ fat, 1 fruit

4 frozen peach slices or ½ large peach, chopped

¼ cup frozen or fresh raspberries

⅓ cup unsweetened pomegranate juice

⅓ cup unsweetened coconut milk or plain coconut-milk kefir

1 scoop vanilla SLIM Protein or Dr. Kellyann–approved protein powder

⅓ cup ice cubes (if not using frozen fruit, use more ice, if desired)

In a blender, puree the peaches, raspberries, pomegranate juice, coconut milk, protein powder, and ice until smooth and frothy, about 1 minute.

## CHAPTER 12

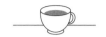

# Make It a 20:

## *Time to Sprinkle a Little Fairy Dust!*

**EARLIER, I TOLD YOU** all about my 80/20 Plan for maintaining your weight loss. On this plan, you'll stick to the basic Bone Broth Diet plan for 80 percent of your meals, and sprinkle a little fairy dust on the rest.

Your 20-percent meals can include pretty much anything from a slice of pizza to a ballpark hot dog. I'll even look the other way if you want to eat a doughnut once a month. At this point, anything's on the table—no pun intended!

However, I do want you to maintain the gains you've worked for so diligently—so here's a little advice for getting the best results during your maintenance phase.

## KEYS TO MAXIMIZING YOUR SUCCESS

While you can eat pretty much any food occasionally on the 80/20 Plan, I recommend centering most of your fairy-dust meals around foods that will help keep your gut glowing, your skin smooth, and your metabolism humming. So I still suggest minimizing dairy, soy, sugar, artificial chemicals, and grains—especially those containing gluten.

Instead, focus on letting favorites like potatoes, rice, and beans back into your diet. And if you aren't ready to give up grains, try quinoa and the other ancient grains I talked about in Chapter 2. They taste great, and they're more in sync with your genetic template than newer grains are.

Also, make sure you continue to load your plate with those nonstarchy veggies. If you want to stay slim, young, and healthy, you need the fiber and nutrients they offer. And don't forget about those fermented veggies like sauerkraut and kimchi, which keep your gut's ecosystem happy.

Finally, keep drinking your bone broth! Now you can use it in new ways; for instance, cooking rice or quinoa, or making mashed potatoes.

## ATTENTION, BAKERS: SWEET TREATS ARE BACK!

On the 80/20 Plan, you can add a dash of sweetness to your life with those healthy sweeteners I talked about in Chapter 2: honey, real maple syrup, blackstrap molasses, and coconut sugar.

These sweeteners are far better for you than sugar because they pack some powerful nutrition. Honey, for instance, is rich in antioxidants and even fights bacteria. Real maple syrup contains more than 50 beneficial compounds. Blackstrap molasses is rich in copper, iron, calcium, vitamin $B_6$, and magnesium. Coconut sugar provides you with potassium, magnesium, zinc, iron, and vitamin C, and it affects your blood sugar less than granulated white sugar does.

You don't want to overload on any of these—after all, you've chased the Sugar Demon out of your life, and you don't want to invite him back in!—but an occasional indulgence is fine. In this chapter, you'll find mouthwatering recipes for cookies, brownies, and other goodies made with nongrain flours and these good-for-you sweeteners.

Are you ready to start sprinkling fairy dust? Then here are some of my favorite "Make it a 20" meals. Ready . . . set . . . sprinkle!

One last note: Since your 80/20 meals aren't part of the basic diet, portion sizes aren't included. However, be sure to stick to the serving sizes I've listed. That way, you can have a little fun without letting those pounds creep back on!

# BLUEBERRY FLAX CARDAMOM MUFFINS

If you're Scandinavian, I'm betting that you already know and love cardamom—a hugely popular spice in Scandinavian countries. This exotic, nutmeg-like spice pairs beautifully with citrus, which is why I've teamed it up here with orange juice and grated orange peel.

PREP TIME: 10 minutes
COOK TIME: 35 minutes
YIELD: 6 servings

- 1 cup almond flour
- 2 tablespoons coconut flour
- 2 tablespoons ground flaxseeds
- 2 teaspoons grated orange peel
- 1 teaspoon baking powder
- ½ teaspoon ground cardamom
- ¼ teaspoon Celtic or pink Himalayan salt
- 1 large egg
- ¼ cup unsweetened plain coconut-milk kefir or coconut milk
- ¼ cup unsweetened applesauce
- 2 tablespoons fresh orange juice
- 2 tablespoons maple syrup
- ½ teaspoon vanilla extract
- ¾ cup frozen unsweetened wild blueberries

Preheat the oven to 350°F. Coat 6 cups of a muffin pan with cooking spray or line with paper liners.

In a large bowl, combine the almond flour, coconut flour, ground flax, orange peel, baking powder, cardamom, and salt.

In a medium bowl, combine the egg, kefir, applesauce, orange juice, maple syrup, and vanilla. Stir the wet ingredients into the flour mixture and mix until just combined. Fold in the blueberries.

Spoon the batter into the prepared muffin cups. Bake until a wooden pick inserted into the center of a muffin comes out clean, about 25 minutes. Cool in the pan for 5 minutes, then remove to a rack to cool completely.

# BREAKFAST CHERRY-ALMOND TEA CAKE

In June or July, when cherries are in season, I always put this cake on my morning menu. It's like summer on a plate!

PREP TIME: 10 minutes
COOK TIME: 40 minutes
YIELD: 12 servings

2 cups almond meal

2 tablespoons arrowroot powder

4 large eggs, separated

⅓ cup honey

½ cup ghee, melted

1 cup cherries, pitted (or thawed, if frozen)

Preheat the oven to 350°F. Coat a 10-inch tart pan with coconut oil spray and line the bottom with a round of parchment paper.

In a large bowl, stir together the almond meal and arrowroot powder. Add the egg yolks, honey, and ghee and mix well to combine. In a separate, clean bowl, with an electric mixer, whip the egg whites until soft peaks form. Fold one-third of the egg whites into the almond mixture, then fold in the remaining egg whites.

Spread the mixture into the prepared pan. Dot the cherries evenly on top of the batter. Bake until golden and firm in the center, 30 to 35 minutes. Cool completely in the pan on a rack before slicing.

# CHICKEN BREASTS STUFFED with MILLET, DRIED FRUIT, and PECANS

Looking for a standout dish for a special occasion? In this fancy recipe, a Mediterranean-style stuffing gets spooned into pockets in chicken breasts, which get pan-fried until golden and then finished off in the oven.

PREP TIME: 10 minutes
COOK TIME: 50 minutes
YIELD: 4 servings

2 cups Chicken Bone Broth (page 65)

½ cup millet

Celtic or pink Himalayan salt

½ cup fresh cilantro or parsley, chopped, plus more for garnish

⅓ cup pecans, chopped

4 unsweetened dried apricot halves or 1 fresh apricot, chopped

2 dried figs or 1 fresh fig, chopped

½ shallot, finely chopped

½ teaspoon ras el hanout (Moroccan seasoning)

4 boneless, skinless chicken breasts (4–5 ounces each)

Freshly ground black pepper

1 tablespoon olive oil

Preheat the oven to 375°F.

In a medium saucepan, bring the bone broth to a boil. Add the millet and ¼ teaspoon salt, cover, reduce the heat to medium-low, and simmer until the millet is tender, 35 to 40 minutes.

Fluff the millet with a fork, then stir in the cilantro, pecans, apricots, figs, shallot, ras el hanout, and a pinch of salt. Set half aside and cover to keep warm.

Cut a lengthwise horizontal slit into the side of the thickest part of each chicken breast, being careful not to poke through the other side. Use the knife to enlarge the pocket, then spoon in 3 to 4 tablespoons stuffing. Season the breasts with salt and pepper.

In a large ovenproof skillet, heat the oil over medium heat. Carefully transfer the stuffed breasts to the skillet. Cook until browned on one side, 3 to 4 minutes, then carefully turn and transfer the skillet to the oven. Bake until a thermometer inserted into the chicken and stuffing registers 165°F and the juices run clear, about 7 minutes.

To serve, sprinkle the chicken with additional chopped cilantro (if desired) and serve with the reserved millet mixture.

# CHILI VERDE

You can make this Southwestern favorite, loaded with chicken, beans, and tomatillos, as mild or as bold as you like. That's why the mouth-burning habanero is optional!

PREP TIME: 15 minutes

COOK TIME: 40 minutes

YIELD: 4 servings

2 tablespoons olive oil

1 large onion, chopped

3 cloves garlic, chopped

1 poblano pepper, seeded and chopped (wear gloves when handling)

1 habanero chile (optional), seeded and chopped (wear gloves when handling)

1 pound ground chicken

1 pound tomatillos, husked, rinsed, and chopped

2 cans (15 ounces each) white beans, rinsed and drained

1 cup Chicken Bone Broth (page 65)

Celtic or pink Himalayan salt and freshly ground black pepper

Cilantro leaves, for garnish

2 cups cooked brown rice

Lime wedges, for serving

In a large pot, heat the oil over medium heat. Add the onion, garlic, poblano, and habanero (if using) and cook until softened, about 8 minutes.

Stir in the ground chicken and cook until no longer pink, about 5 minutes. Add the tomatillos, beans, broth, and salt and pepper to taste and bring to a simmer. Cook until thickened, about 20 minutes.

Garnish with cilantro and serve over brown rice, with lime wedges on the side.

# SLOW COOKER OSSO BUCO

Osso buco is Italian for "bone with a hole," referring to the marrow holes in the centers of veal shanks. Cooking the shanks for hours makes them fork-tender; topped with the rich braising sauce, they're soul-satisfying.

PREP TIME: 20 minutes
COOK TIME: 8 hours 30 minutes
YIELD: 4 servings

4 veal shanks (1½–2 inches thick), trimmed and tied around the circumference with kitchen string

Celtic or pink Himalayan salt and freshly ground black pepper

½ cup coconut flour

2 tablespoons olive oil or tallow

1 large onion, finely chopped

2 ribs celery, finely chopped

1 carrot, finely chopped

1 parsnip, finely chopped

1 teaspoon fresh thyme leaves (from 4 sprigs)

1 teaspoon fresh rosemary leaves, chopped

1 bay leaf

1 tablespoon tomato paste

Season the shanks liberally with salt and pepper. Put the coconut flour in a shallow dish and dust both sides of each shank in the flour. In a large skillet, heat the oil over medium heat. Add the shanks and sear until a deep brown crust forms on both sides, about 4 minutes per side. Transfer the shanks to a slow cooker, nestling so they fit in one layer.

Increase the heat under the skillet to medium-high. Add the onion, celery, carrot, parsnip, thyme, rosemary, bay leaf, and ½ teaspoon each salt and pepper. Cook, stirring frequently, until the vegetables start to soften and brown, about 6 minutes. Add the tomato paste and stir to distribute, about 2 minutes. Add the broth and scrape up the browned bits from the bottom of the skillet. Cook until the broth is thoroughly heated through, 1 to 2 minutes. Stir in the vinegar.

Pour the contents of the skillet over the shanks in the slow cooker. Cover and cook on low until the meat is very tender and falling off the bone, 7½ to 8 hours.

In a small bowl, combine the parsley, garlic, lemon peel, and a healthy pinch of salt. Cover and refrigerate until ready to serve.

Transfer the shanks to a platter and remove the strings. Carefully drain the contents of the slow cooker through a sieve into a bowl, reserving the liquid and adding the solids to the plate with the shanks (discard the bay leaf). Cover with foil to keep warm.

1½ cups Italian Beef Bone Broth (page 75)

2 teaspoons balsamic vinegar

¼ cup fresh flat-leaf parsley leaves, finely chopped

2 cloves garlic, minced

2 teaspoons grated lemon peel

8 ounces brown rice noodles or quinoa noodles

Transfer the strained cooking liquid to a skillet. Bring to a boil over high heat and cook until the liquid is reduced and achieves a gravy-like consistency, about 5 minutes.

Meanwhile, prepare the noodles according to the package directions.

To serve, arrange the noodles in large pasta bowls or on plates. Set the veal with vegetables on top of the noodles. Top with the sauce and garnish with the parsley mixture. Serve with a spoon to scrape out the marrow from the bones.

# TURKEY TV DINNER

Curl up on the couch, turn on your favorite show, and enjoy this fun blast from the past. My recipe remake is healthy from start to finish, while featuring all of the classic ingredients you love—including a luscious gravy.

PREP TIME: 15 minutes

COOK TIME: 1 hour

YIELD: 4 servings

1 bone-in, skin-on turkey breast (1–1½ pounds)

1 tablespoon olive oil

Celtic or pink Himalayan salt and freshly ground black pepper

2 pounds russet potatoes, peeled and coarsely chopped

¼ cup ghee, melted

½ pound green beans

1 cup Chicken Bone Broth (page 65)

2 tablespoons arrowroot powder

Preheat the oven to 450°F.

Rub the turkey breast all over with the oil and season with salt and pepper. Place skin side up in a small baking pan. Place in the oven and immediately reduce the temperature to 350°F. Roast until a thermometer inserted in the thickest part registers 165°F and the juices run clear, about 45 minutes.

Meanwhile, in a medium pot of boiling water, cook the potatoes until cooked through, about 15 minutes. Drain and mash with the ghee and season to taste with salt and pepper. Set aside and keep warm.

In a medium pot fitted with a steamer basket, bring 1 inch of water to a boil. Add the green beans to the basket, cover, and steam until bright green and tender, about 5 minutes. Set aside and keep warm.

When the turkey is done, remove it from the pan and set aside. Put the pan on the stovetop over medium-high heat. Add the broth and bring to a boil, using a spatula to scrape up any browned bits on the bottom of the pan. In a small bowl, stir the arrowroot powder with 2 tablespoons water until dissolved. Remove the pan from the heat, stir in the arrowroot, season to taste with salt and pepper, and whisk until thickened.

To serve, slice the turkey breast. Divide the turkey, mashed potatoes, and green beans among 4 plates, and serve with the gravy. Rectangular, sectioned plates are optional!

# KOREAN RICE BOWL

This spicy meal-in-a-bowl features beef, eggs, veggies, and kimchi—with an added dash of hot-peper sauce, if you're feeling brave!—all served over a scoop of brown rice.

PREP TIME: 15 minutes
COOK TIME: 30 minutes
YIELD: 4 servings

- 2 tablespoons coconut aminos
- 1 teaspoon toasted sesame oil
- 1 teaspoon grated fresh ginger
- 1 clove garlic, minced
- 1 pound beef sirloin, trimmed
- 1 cup brown rice
- 3 medium carrots, thinly sliced
- 4 ounces shiitake mushrooms, stems discarded, caps sliced
- 5 ounces baby spinach
- 2 teaspoons olive oil
- 4 large eggs
- 1 cup kimchi
- Gluten-free hot-pepper sauce (optional)

In a large bowl, stir together the coconut aminos, sesame oil, ginger, and garlic. Add the beef and set aside to marinate while you cook the rice and vegetables.

Cook the rice according to package directions. Set aside and keep warm.

In a medium pot fitted with a steamer basket, bring 1 inch of water to a boil. Steam the vegetables separately in the basket: carrots until crisp-tender, shiitakes until softened, and spinach until wilted and bright green, about 2 minutes each. Set each aside and keep warm.

In a large skillet, heat 1 teaspoon of the olive oil over medium heat until shimmering. Remove the steak from the marinade (discard the marinade) and cook, turning halfway through, until a thermometer inserted in the center registers 160°F for medium, 8 minutes (or until desired doneness). Rest the steak for 10 minutes before slicing very thinly.

Wipe out the skillet, heat the remaining 1 teaspoon olive oil, and cook the eggs sunny-side up, about 2 minutes.

To serve, divide the rice among 4 bowls. Top each with the steamed vegetables, kimchi, beef, and 1 egg. Serve with hot-pepper sauce on the side, if desired.

# SHEPHERD'S PIE

Alternating slices of russet potato and sweet potato create a pretty topping for this rustic dish. The filling stars lamb braised with wine and seasoned with rosemary and garlic.

PREP TIME: 10 minutes
COOK TIME: 55 minutes
YIELD: 4 servings

1 tablespoon olive oil

1 medium onion, finely chopped

Celtic or pink Himalayan salt

1½ teaspoons finely chopped fresh rosemary

2 cloves garlic, minced

1 pound ground lamb

⅓ cup red wine

1 can (14.5 ounces) diced tomatoes, drained

⅓ cup Chicken Bone Broth (page 65) or Beef Bone Broth (page 67)

1 tablespoon tomato paste

¼ cup chopped fresh flat-leaf parsley leaves

Freshly ground black pepper

1 large russet potato, scrubbed and thinly sliced

1 large sweet potato, scrubbed and thinly sliced

2 tablespoons ghee, melted

In a large, deep skillet or Dutch oven, heat the oil over medium-high heat. Add the onion, season with a pinch of salt, and cook, stirring frequently, until soft and light golden brown, about 8 minutes. Add the rosemary and garlic and cook until fragrant, about 1 minute. Add the meat and cook, breaking it up with a wooden spoon, until no longer pink, about 5 minutes. Increase the heat, add the wine, and bring to a boil. Add the tomatoes, broth, and tomato paste and bring to a simmer. Cook, stirring occasionally, until the liquid has reduced to a sauce consistency and coats the meat, about 20 minutes.

Preheat the oven to 400°F.

Let the lamb mixture cool slightly and stir in the parsley. Season to taste with salt and pepper. Pour the lamb into an 8 × 8-inch baking dish.

Toss the potatoes with the ghee and shingle over the lamb, alternating between white potato and sweet potato. Sprinkle with salt and pepper and bake until the potatoes are tender and golden, about 20 minutes.

# SEAFOOD SOFRITO

A sofrito is a mix of garlic, tomato, onions, and olive oil that forms the base for a dish—in this case, a combo of clams, mussels, and scallops. I've added a bell pepper for even more veggie goodness.

PREP TIME: 15 minutes
COOK TIME: 35 minutes
YIELD: 4 servings

3 tablespoons extra-virgin olive oil

Pinch of saffron threads

1½ cups brown basmati rice

Celtic or pink Himalayan salt

1 medium yellow onion, finely chopped

1 small green bell pepper, finely chopped

3 cloves garlic, minced

½ teaspoon dried oregano

½ teaspoon ground cumin

Freshly ground black pepper

½ cup dry white wine

1 can (8 ounces) no-sugar-added tomato sauce

½ pound littleneck clams, scrubbed

½ pound mussels, scrubbed and debearded (see Tip)

½ pound bay scallops

1 large lemon, cut into wedges

In a 4-quart saucepan, heat 1 tablespoon of the oil and the saffron over medium-high heat until the saffron is sizzling. Add the rice and stir to coat. Add 3½ cups water and a pinch of salt and bring to a boil. Boil for 1 minute. Reduce the heat to a gentle simmer, stir once, cover, and cook until all of the water has been absorbed and the rice is tender, about 35 minutes.

Meanwhile, in a 12-inch skillet, heat the remaining 2 tablespoons oil over medium heat. Add the onion, bell pepper, and garlic and cook, stirring, until the vegetables are soft, about 8 minutes. Stir in the oregano, cumin, and ½ teaspoon each salt and pepper. Add the wine and simmer until reduced by half, about 3 minutes. Stir in the tomato sauce and 1 cup water and bring to a simmer. Reduce the heat to low, cover, and cook until slightly thickened, about 5 minutes.

Nestle in the clams, cover the pan, and cook for 5 minutes. Stir in the mussels and scallops, cover, and cook until all the shells have opened, about 5 minutes more. (Discard any shells that do not open.)

Transfer the rice to a large platter, top with the seafood mixture, and sprinkle with more pepper. Serve immediately with lemon wedges.

TIP: *The beard is the mossy-looking bit that hangs off the mussel at the hinge, where the two shells join. It's not inedible, but it is a bit unpleasant. Not every mussel will have a beard, and all it takes is a little tug to pull it free. Tug toward the hinge of the mussel, and give it a wiggle to pull it free.*

# VEGETABLE CURRY

This scrumptious curry showcases many of my favorite super-foods, from bone broth and coconut milk to healthy spices and more than half a dozen fruits and veggies. Brown rice makes it a one-pan meal.

PREP TIME: 15 minutes
COOK TIME: 25 minutes
YIELD: 4 servings

2 tablespoons coconut oil or ghee

½ yellow onion, finely chopped

1 small sweet potato, peeled and chopped

1 carrot, finely chopped

3 cloves garlic, minced

1 tablespoon grated fresh ginger

1 tablespoon curry powder or hot Madras curry powder (see Tip)

½ teaspoon ground cardamom

1 can (14.5 ounces) diced tomatoes

1½ cups Chicken Bone Broth (page 65) or Asian Chicken Bone Broth (page 72)

¾ cup canned coconut milk, well stirred

½ teaspoon Celtic or pink Himalayan salt

¼ teaspoon freshly ground black pepper

1 cup brown basmati rice

2 cups baby spinach

2 tablespoons chopped fresh cilantro, for serving

Lime wedges, for serving

In a large skillet with a lid, melt the coconut oil over medium heat. Add the onion, sweet potato, and carrot and cook, stirring, until softened, 8 minutes.

Add the garlic, ginger, curry powder, and cardamom and cook until fragrant, about 1 minute. Add the tomatoes with their juice, broth, coconut milk, salt, and pepper, stirring to combine. Bring to a simmer. Stir in the rice, reduce the heat, cover, and cook until the flavors meld and the rice is nearly done, about 10 minutes.

Stir in the spinach, cover, and continue cooking until the sauce is heated through and the rice is tender, 3 to 5 minutes more.

Serve sprinkled with cilantro, with lime wedges on the side.

TIP: *Using hot Madras curry powder will add more heat to this dish.*

# CHOCOLATE HAZELNUT PIE

Reminiscent of pecan pie, this melt-in-your-mouth dessert is simple as—well, pie! Just whirl everything in your food processor, and you're all set.

PREP TIME: 15 minutes
COOK TIME: 1 hour
YIELD: 8 servings

**For the crust:**

- ¾ cup hazelnuts, skins removed (see Tip)
- ¼ cup coconut oil, melted
- 1 cup coconut flour
- 2 tablespoons maple syrup
- ¼ teaspoon Celtic or pink Himalayan salt

**For the filling:**

- 8 ounces pitted dates (about 2 cups)
- ½ cup coconut oil, melted
- 1 cup unsweetened cocoa powder
- ¼ cup maple syrup
- 1 teaspoon vanilla extract
- Toasted hazelnuts, crushed, for garnish (optional)

*For the crust:* Preheat the oven to 400°F.

In a food processor, pulse the hazelnuts into a coarse powder. Add the coconut oil, coconut flour, maple syrup, and salt and pulse until the mixture holds together. Press into the bottom and up the sides of a 9-inch pie plate. Pierce the bottom of the crust all over with a fork and bake until the edges are browned, 8 to 10 minutes. Cool completely.

*For the filling:* Soak the dates in boiling water for 15 minutes. Drain off the water and add the dates to a food processor. Pulse a few times to break up the dates, then add the coconut oil, cocoa, maple syrup, and vanilla. Process until the mixture is mostly smooth, 1 to 2 minutes. Spread into the cooled crust and refrigerate for 30 minutes before serving.

Garnish with crushed toasted hazelnuts, if desired.

**TIP:** *To remove hazelnut skins, preheat an oven to 350°F. Spread the hazelnuts on a large rimmed baking sheet and toast until the skins begin to pull away from the nut, about 8 minutes. Transfer to a large kitchen towel and use the towel to rub all the skins off.*

# DR. KELLYANN'S OMG CHOCOLATE CHIP COOKIES

These cookies are so delicious that when I give them out as holiday gifts, everyone demands the recipe. For a change of pace, make them with chocolate chunks instead.

PREP TIME: 10 minutes plus refrigerating time
COOK TIME: 10 minutes

YIELD: 12 cookies

1½ cups almond flour

¼ teaspoon baking soda

¼ teaspoon sea salt

2 tablespoons coconut oil, melted

½ teaspoon vanilla extract

¼ cup honey

1 egg, at room temperature

¾ cup chocolate chips (see Tip)

In a large bowl, combine the almond flour, baking soda, and salt.

In a separate bowl, beat the coconut oil, vanilla, honey, and egg. Add the wet ingredients to the dry ingredients and mix well to combine. Mix in the chocolate chips. Cover and refrigerate the cookie dough for 30 minutes.

Preheat the oven to 350°F. Line a baking sheet with parchment paper.

Roll the dough into 12 balls and arrange them on the baking sheet. Bake for 5 minutes. Remove the pan from the oven and flatten the cookies slightly with the back of a spoon. Put them back in the oven for about 5 minutes more, or until they look done. If you like soft and chewy cookies, take them out as soon as they start to turn golden brown.

Remove from the oven and let the cookies remain on the pan for 1 minute before transferring them to racks to cool.

TIP: *Try the Enjoy Life brand chocolate chips—they're dairy-, soy-, and nut-free.*

# COCONUT CAKE with DEEP CHOCOLATE FROSTING

This is one of my favorite special-occasion desserts. Serve it at a birthday party or a baby shower, and no one will guess that it's actually healthy!

PREP TIME: 5 minutes
COOK TIME: 45 minutes
YIELD: 12 servings

**For the cake:**

- 1 cup coconut flour
- ½ teaspoon Celtic or pink Himalayan salt
- ½ teaspoon baking soda
- 8 large eggs
- ½ cup coconut oil, melted
- ½ cup maple syrup
- 2 teaspoons vanilla extract

**For the frosting:**

- ½ cup unsweetened cocoa powder
- ¼ cup coconut oil, melted
- 2 tablespoons maple syrup
- ¼ teaspoon vanilla extract
- Pinch of Celtic or pink Himalayan salt

*For the cake:* Preheat the oven to 350°F. Coat an 8-inch round cake pan with coconut oil spray and line the bottom with a round of parchment paper.

In a medium bowl, stir together the coconut flour, salt, and baking soda. In a stand mixer fitted with the paddle attachment, mix the eggs, coconut oil, maple syrup, and vanilla until well combined. Add the dry ingredients and mix well, making sure there are no lumps.

Spread the batter into the prepared pan and bake until golden and brown around the edges, 25 to 30 minutes. Let cool in the pan for 10 minutes, then turn out onto a rack to cool completely.

*For the frosting:* In a bowl, stir together the cocoa, coconut oil, maple syrup, vanilla, and salt until smooth. Spread on the cooled cake.

# BLACK FOREST BROWNIES

Chocolate and cherries team up in a gooey, decadent treat. These brownies taste *way* too good to be good for you . . . and yet they are!

PREP TIME: 10 minutes
COOK TIME: 50 minutes
YIELD: 16 servings

10 ounces frozen unsweetened black or sweet cherries (2 cups)

¼ teaspoon almond extract

8 ounces unsweetened chocolate (100% cacao), chopped

½ cup ghee or coconut oil

⅓ cup maple syrup

¼ cup unsweetened almond milk

1 teaspoon vanilla extract

4 large eggs

¼ cup ground flaxseeds

2 tablespoons coconut flour

½ teaspoon Celtic or pink Himalayan salt

Preheat the oven to 350°F. Grease an 8 × 8-inch baking pan.

In a medium saucepan, combine the cherries, 2 tablespoons water, and the almond extract. Simmer over medium heat, mashing with a potato masher when the cherries are thawed, until thick and syrupy, about 10 minutes. Set aside.

Meanwhile, in a medium bowl set over a pot of simmering water (but not touching the water), melt the chocolate, ghee, and maple syrup, stirring to combine. Remove from the heat and cool briefly.

To the chocolate, whisk in the almond milk and vanilla, then the eggs, one at a time, until thoroughly incorporated. Whisk in the ground flax, coconut flour, and salt until just combined. Pour into the prepared pan, spreading evenly.

Dollop the cherry mixture around the surface of the brownies and use a spoon or knife to swirl. Bake until a wooden pick inserted into the center comes out clean or with a few moist crumbs, about 25 minutes. Let cool in the pan for 10 minutes before cutting and serving.

# JOIN THE FUN!

The Bone Broth Diet official hashtag is #BoneBrothDiet. Add this hashtag to any posting you do, and my social media team or others online will be able to connect with you. Also, use #BoneBrothRecipes to get more fantastic recipe ideas.

In addition, look for me on Facebook at DrKellyann/Facebook, where you'll find a community of more than 100,000 people. It's one of the most fun, exciting communities anywhere online—be a part of it!

You can hashtag on Twitter @DrKellyann and on Instagram @DrKellyannPetrucci.

# APPENDIX

# *Measurement Tracker*

**FILL OUT THIS FORM** before and after your diet so you can quantify your results. I also suggest taking before-and-after photos of yourself from different angles.

| BEGINNING OF THE DIET | | | | | COMPLETION OF THE DIET | | | | |
|---|---|---|---|---|---|---|---|---|---|
| Current Weight | | | | | Current Weight | | | | |
| Current Measurements | | | | | Current Measurements | | | | |
| Biceps | Chest | Waist | Hips | Thighs | Biceps | Chest | Waist | Hips | Thighs |
| | | | | | | | | | |
| Current BMI | | | | | Current BMI | | | | |

**TO CALCULATE YOUR BMI (BODY MASS INDEX):**

**Measure your height in inches.** To do this, stand against a wall and use a pencil to make a mark at the top of your head.

**Take your height in inches and square the number.** (Multiply the number of inches by itself.)

**Divide your weight in pounds by your height in inches squared.**

**Multiply the answer by 703.** This is your body mass index. While this number isn't infallible, it can give you a rough idea of the amount of body fat you have. Here's a guide you can use.

| BMI | WEIGHT |
|---|---|
| Below 18.5 | Underweight |
| 18.5–24.9 | Normal or healthy weight |
| 25.0–29.9 | Overweight |
| 30.0 and above | Obese |

# BEFORE-AND-AFTER MEDICAL TESTS

If you're interested in how the diet affects your overall health, ask your doctor to do tests before and after the diet and record this information at each point.

- Your blood pressure
- Your blood sugar levels
- Your levels of C-reactive protein
- Your cholesterol and triglyceride levels
- Your pH (acid-base balance)

# ENDNOTES

## CHAPTER 1

1   Alice G. Walton, "Why Oreos Are as Addictive as Cocaine to Your Brain," Forbes, October 16, 2013.

2   David Sack, "Kids on Sweets: Are We Raising a Generation of Sugar Addicts?" Huffington Post, November 6, 2013.

3   M. C. Hochberg et al., "Combined Chondroitin Sulfate and Glucosamine for Painful Knee Osteoarthritis: A Multicentre, Randomised, Double-Blind, Non-Inferiority Trial versus Celecoxib," *Annals of the Rheumatic Diseases* (January 14, 2015), ard.bmj.com/content/early/2015/01/14/annrheumdis-2014-206792.full.

4   M. Tanaka, Y. Koyama, and Y. Nomura, "Effects of Collagen Peptide Ingestion on UV-B-Induced Skin Damage," *Bioscience, Biotechnology, and Biochemistry* 73, no. 4 (April 23, 2009): 930-2.

## CHAPTER 3

1   K. Esposito et al., "Inflammatory Cytokine Concentrations Are Acutely Increased by Hyperglycemia in Humans: Role of Oxidative Stress," *Circulation* 106, no. 16 (October 15, 2002): 2067–72.

2   F. W. Danby, "Nutrition and Aging Skin: Sugar and Glycation," *Clinical Dermatology* 28, no. 4 (July–August 2010): 409–11.

3   Amanda MacMillan, "This is How Sugar May 'Fuel' Cancer Cells," Fox News Health, July 2, 2016.

4   Julie Corliss, "Eating Too Much Added Sugar Increases the Risk of Dying with Heart Disease," Harvard Health Blog, December 1, 2015.

5   E. R. Shell, "Artificial Sweeteners May Change Our Gut Bacteria in Dangerous Ways," *Scientific American*, April 1, 2015.

6   D. Vergano, "Study: Artificial Sweeteners May Trigger Blood Sugar Risks," *National Geographic*, September 17, 2014.

7   L. Conti, "Artificial Sweeteners Confound the Brain; May Lead to Diet Disaster," *Scientific American*, June 1, 2008.

8   K. de Punder and L. Pruimboom, "The Dietary Intake of Wheat and Other Cereal Grains and Their Role in Inflammation," *Nutrients* 5 no. 3 (March 2013): 771–87.

9   Jenn Harris, "Cheese Really Is Crack. Study Reveals Cheese Is as Addictive as Drugs," *Los Angeles Times*, October 22, 2015.

10   L. Tran et al., "Soy Extracts Suppressed Iodine Uptake and Stimulated the Production of Autoimmunogen in Rat Thyrocytes," *Experimental Biology and Medicine* 238, no. 6 (June 2013): 623–30.

11   *Bulletin de l'Office Federal de la Sante Publique*, no. 28, July 20, 1992.

12   EWG's Dirty Dozen Guide to Food Additives, ewg.org/research/ewg-s-dirty-dozen -guide-food-additives.

13   Ibid.

14   Ibid.

15   Ibid.

## CHAPTER 6

1   C.N. Blesso, C.J. Andersen, J. Barona, J.S. Volek, and M.L. Fernandez, "Whole Egg Consumption Improves Lipoprotein Profiles and Insulin Sensitivity to a Greater Extent Than Yolk-Free Egg Substitute in Individuals with Metabolic Syndrome," *Metabolism* 62, no. 3 (March 2013): 400–10.

2   Ben Tinker, "Cholesterol in Food Not a Concern, New Report Says," CNN, February 19, 2015.

## CHAPTER 7

1   Mark Bittman, "Butter Is Back," *New York Times*, March 25, 2014.

## CHAPTER 9

1   J. E. Flood and B. J. Rolls, "Soup Preloads in a Variety of Forms Reduce Meal Energy Intake," *Appetite* 49, no. 3 (November 2007): 626–34.

# INDEX

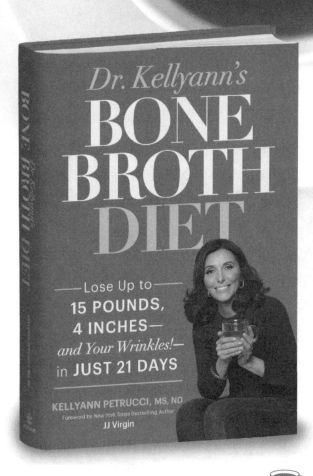

# YOUR SECRET WEAPON for FAST, HUNGER-FREE WEIGHT LOSS

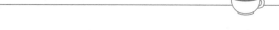

Celebrities and athletes are hooked on it, morning talk-show hosts are raving about it, and foodies everywhere are making it in their own kitchens.

Bone broth isn't just broth. It isn't just soup. It's concentrated healing.

Packed with fat-burning nutrients, skin-tightening collagen components, and gut-healing and anti-inflammatory properties, this magical food is the key to looking and feeling younger than ever before.

With DR. KELLYANN'S BONE BROTH DIET, you can lose up to 15 pounds, achieve more youthful-looking skin, and fight cravings in just 21 days.

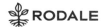